The BIRTH BOOK

Your guide to a positive birth experience

The information provided in this book is for educational and general purposes only. It is not intended to be a substitute for professional medical advice and should not be relied on as health or personal advice. It is important that you always seek the guidance of your doctor or other qualified health professional with any questions you may have regarding your health or a medical condition.

First published 2022

Big Sky Publishing Pty Ltd

PO Box 303, Newport, NSW 2106, Australia

Phone: 1300 364 611

Fax: (61 2) 9918 2396

Email: info@bigskypublishing.com.au

Web: www.bigskypublishing.com.au

Cover design and typesetting: Think Productions

Proudly printed and bound in China

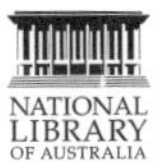

A catalogue record for this book is available from the National Library of Australia

For Cataloguing-in-Publication entry see National Library of Australia.

The BIRTH BOOK

Your guide to a positive birth experience

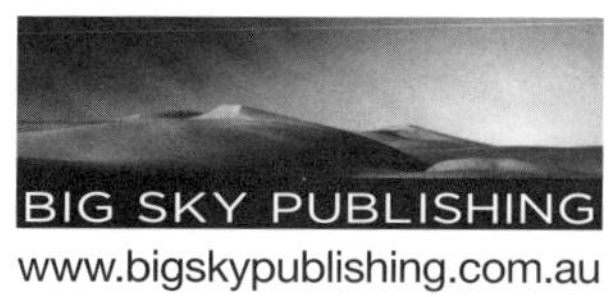

PROF STEPHEN TONG

To Carol, Katrina, Laura and Poppy,
and to the many whose births I have been privileged to attend.

Contents

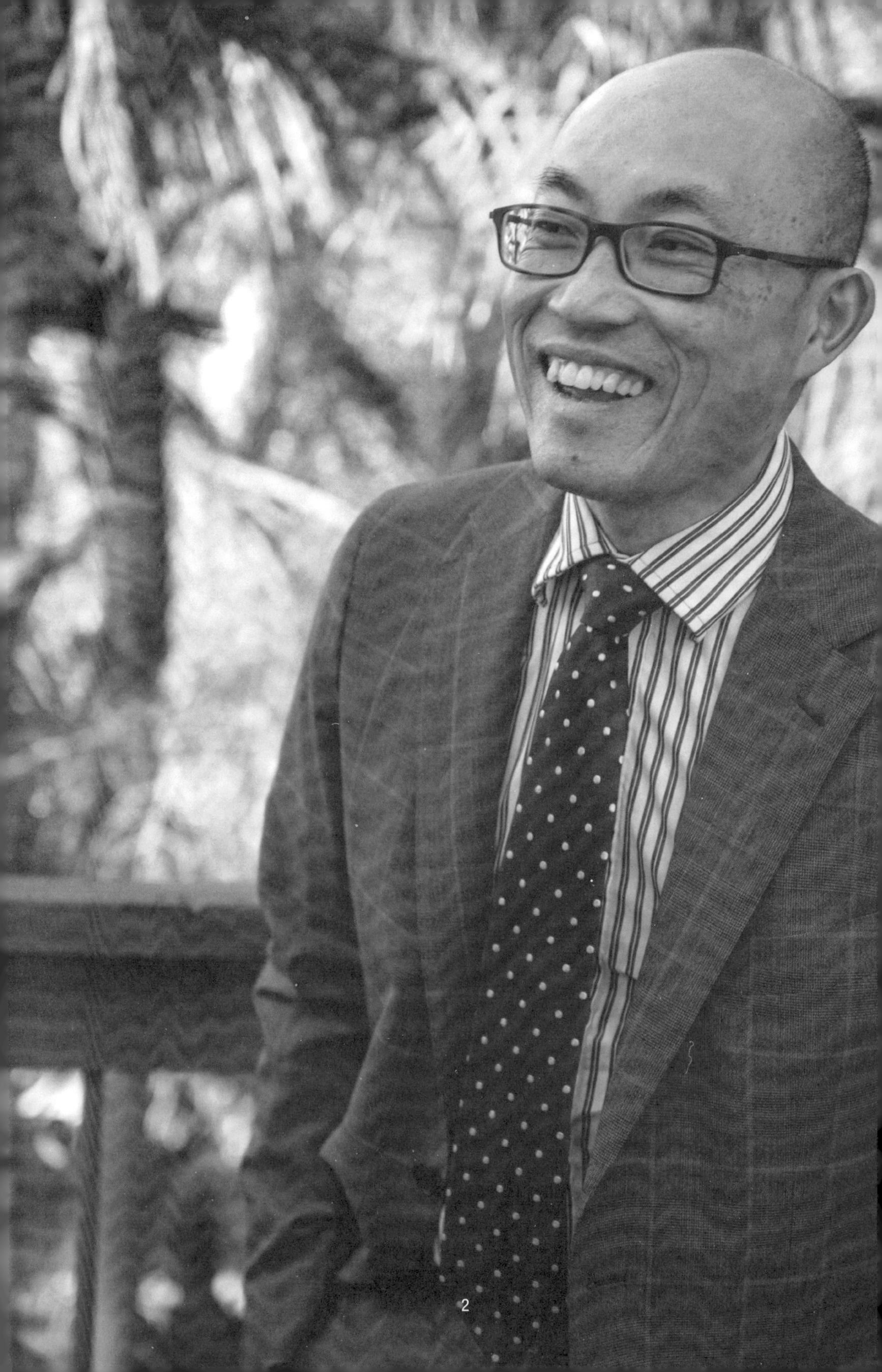

About the Author

Stephen Tong is among Australia's top Professors of Obstetrics and Gynaecology who has dedicated his life to finding better ways of ensuring safer motherhood and birth.

As a specialist obstetrician, he has been providing pregnancy care for two decades. Stephen has personally assisted in the birth of thousands of babies. He continues to practise his craft at Mercy Hospital for Women, one of the leading academic maternity hospitals in Australia. There, he also trains obstetric specialists of the future.

As a research academic, Stephen is widely known internationally within his research field. Leading a large team of scientists and clinical researchers, Stephen is chasing discoveries to make pregnancy safer.

Stephen is one of the lead investigators running several clinical trials across the world testing new treatments to tackle major complications of pregnancy. Many of these treatments were originally discovered by Stephen's laboratory team in Melbourne before being launched into international clinical trials.

He has authored over 180 scientific papers, many of which have been published in prestigious international journals. In recognition of his research achievements, has received three major national awards from the National Health and Medical Research Council of Australia (NHMRC).

Connect with Stephen:

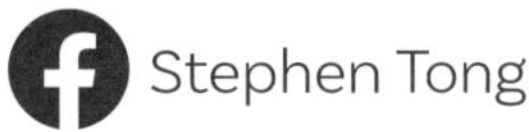

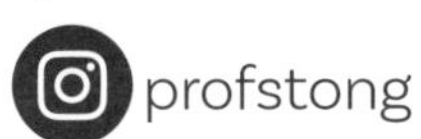

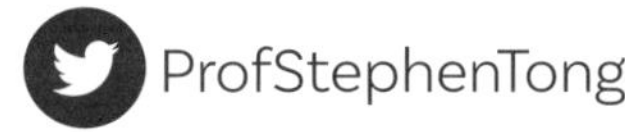

Praise for *The Birth Book*

"Finally a birthing book that delivers facts in a non-judgemental, warm and witty way. Stephen's unique way of approaching birth, one that is steeped in science but swathed in soul, is an uplifting one that brings joy and laughter instead of fear and tears to the birthing suite."

Dani Venn, celebrity chef, mum of two

"Empowering yourself with the knowledge needed to navigate childbirth. This book is fun, easy to read, educational and will have you laughing and even crying sometimes. An absolute must read for expecting parents and their support team."

Associate Professor Cathy Cluver – pregnancy researcher, mum of three

"This book is going to save so much googling time for women before their birth. It's all there, everything you need to know, with a bit of kookiness along the way. I really think it will help so many anxious women feel more prepared for their birth and give them the best gift ever–enjoying the best day of their life, with no worries."

Kristie Gatanios, professional singer and teacher, mum of one

"A fascinating, refreshing, easy read about the final step on the journey to motherhood. This book includes everything I wish I knew about birthing before I arrived in the birthing suite. Humourous anecdotes coupled with a clear, unbiased and supportive view on what to expect make this a must-read for every Australian soon-to-be mum and her birthing team."

Sarah Ng, instructional designer, mum of three

“An informative and entertaining ‘road-map’ towards birth and the many different routes the journey might take you on. A must read for the pregnant person as they head towards delivery day”

Associate Professor Tu’uhevaha Kaitu’u-Lino,
pregnancy researcher, mum of four

"A humorous and informative account of labour and birth. A realistic account exposing the truth behind one of the most intimate experiences in human life. Prepare yourself for a brilliantly written journey of laughter and enlightenment."

Alison Abboud, midwife

“It’s like no book that I read before the birth of my three children, and without a doubt the one book that I needed. It’s a raw unbridled look at the wonder of childbirth that will empower and prepare any expecting mother.”

Melissa Wilson, teacher, mum of three

“Hugely informative, witty and compassionate, this book completely demystified birth. I was walked through every step of labour including what happens when things don’t go quite to plan, and what my options are along the way. Most importantly, this book is free from judgement and opinion, offering only decades of experience and easy to understand evidence.”

Dr Roxanne Hastie, pregnancy researcher, mum of one

“Filled with Stephen’s unique wit and humour, *The Birth Book* presents a comprehensive and evidenced-based journey into labour and birth that is an enjoyable and easy read.”

Alex Roddy Mitchell, midwife

Foreword

Welcome to *The Birth Book!* If you have picked this up, it is probably because you- or someone dear to you- is approaching the time of birth. Congratulations! This is an incredibly exciting time in your life. The arrival of a baby heralds an exciting new chapter for everyone in your 'village'. Families and friends stand together with new parents in a shared vision: that love will surround our children all their lives, that good fortune and health will follow them, that we will help launch them into a life of unlimited possibility, that we – through them – will leave this world better than we found it.

Which brings us to the all-important launch pad. Few of us will experience the astronaut's walk to the Kennedy Space Centre launch pad at Cape Canaveral, but many women approaching the day of birth can probably relate to the mixture of intense excitement and nervousness. The sharpened focus. The comfort of customs and rituals that tether us to what makes meaning for us. The immeasurable value of your faithful flight crew on the day and your wider support crew on the ground. But the other thing that can help to ensure this is less of a 'white knuckle ride' is knowledge of what's going on, and trust in the team looking after you. In the launch pad of the birthing suite, this is the midwives, nurses and doctors, and our sole job is to take care of you all – mother, baby and family. To put you at ease. To share with you what's happening and why. To ensure no one is left behind. In short, to ensure a safe and happy birth day.

If this resonates with you, then Professor Stephen Tong's book will hit the mark. Stephen is a highly experienced obstetrician, who I have had the pleasure of working with in the public and private sector over many years in Melbourne, Australia. He is also one of our nation's finest researchers. He has dedicated his life to discovering new and better ways of ensuring safer motherhood and the best possible start to life. He has made world leading discoveries into some of the most perilous complications of pregnancy – stillbirth, preeclampsia, ectopic pregnancy and others. It is true that not all heroes wear capes.

Stephen also has an uncanny ability to distill the essence of a clinical or research problem, and explain it in a thoughtful, kind and wise way that makes sense – peppered with (sometimes quirky but always illustrative!) anecdotes. This is the real art of the clinician or academic – to bring others along with you. I will often walk past his office where he will be shaping a PhD student's research presentation and hear him say, 'You need to tell the story so your grandmother will understand it'. It misses the point if our research or education is impenetrable to the people we are trying to empower and help.

It is this philosophy he has brought to *The Birth Book*. Pregnant women, together with their partners and support team, are bombarded with a lot of information about birth, but the challenge for many is to make sense of it all. This book picks some of this information apart, and then knits it back together into a short, digestible companion for labour and birth. Of course, this garment is not a 'one size fits all'. Nothing can replace the individualized advice and recommendations for you, your baby and circumstance. But this book gives you an important place from which to start the conversation. Here Stephen walks you through the stages of labour and birth, and how we keep mum and baby safe. He explains exactly how different forms of pain relief work so you can help decide what might be best for you. He guides you through the evidence so you can understand – and share in – the clinical decision making that surrounds induction of labour and assisted birth, including caesarean section. He also takes you down some of the roads less travelled in the birthing suite like heavy bleeding after childbirth, so you know how the expert team in Mission Control will spring into action if needed. He might be your invisible partner on the big day, quietly saying, 'Remember we talked about this? This is all OK'.

Importantly, he has presented this in a way that is both calm and informative. We are living through a strange time in history, where information sharing about COVID-19 has made us all armchair experts in pandemic epidemiology, aerosol transmission and the nuances of vaccine effectiveness. Like me, you probably have wise, trusted sources to whom you turn for balanced scientific information – free of political bias, hysteria, hidden agendas and baseless conspiracy theories. Such a source is *The Birth Book*. Your 'access all areas' backstage pass for what goes on behind the birthing suite doors. It is the balanced, 'expert in your pocket' for the big day who – along with wonderful midwives, doctors and childbirth educators- will shepherd you through.

Of course, I'm sure the moment of rocket launch is incomparable to the magic of space travel. The richness that you, your partner, family, customs and traditions bring to your birth and parenting is immeasurable. None of us can replace or replicate it. Ensure this is all part of your birth plan, too. It is your fingerprints, not ours, that belong on your baby's head. Our role – and the intention of this book – is simply to partner with you for the big day: to share our language and customs, to make the birthing suite, its people and practices a warm and familiar place. To provide a confident 'go for launch'. I wish you the most wonderful birth day, and joys untold in your yet-to-be-charted voyage of parenting.

Sue Walker, AO
Professor, Obstetrician, Maternal-Fetal Medicine Specialist

Introduction

Which day was the most important day of your life? The most memorable? If you ask a mum, the day she gave birth is going to rank highly. For many, it'll top the list; placed above her 21st birthday bash (fogged by alcohol), the elation of graduation day, or even that dreamy tropical holiday where she impulsively offered a sip of her tangy strawberry daiquiri to a lonesome stranger, now her loving life partner.

For those who have opted to marry giving birth is likely to be up there with the day of their wedding. And that would be a fair call. Both days, highly memorable, ink permanent spots on the rest of her life. One unites them with a life partner to face the world. The other brings the joy – and challenges – of a child to shape, love and nurture.

Both an upcoming wedding and looming childbirth can be anticipated months before (barring hasty decisions in Vegas by couples swept up in the moment of glitz, cheap beer, and a noisy lights and sirens win at the slot machines). It is therefore a touch curious that these impending occasions are approached so differently.

Courtesy of endless evenings, late nights and weekends consumed by meticulous planning, a bride-to-be is going to know a lot about her wedding well in advance. To the minute detail. She'll know what will be uttered at the ceremony (to the word), be affectionately familiar with every microscopic detail of the ring that will soon adorn her finger (dollar amount and probably the clarity scale of every tiny rock embedded within the glinting band), and exactly where everyone will sit at the reception (with particular thought invested into placing her future mother-in-law). She will know exactly what meals will be served, chosen after much indecision and angst from a delectable listing, which is a little ironic because she is going to be too busy to taste any of it while it is still warm and on the right side of tasty.

In contrast, many will face the day of childbirth knowing a good deal less about what's in store. They may be aware – with some trepidation – that labour will hurt and that at some point they'll need to push hard. Really hard (this is, in fact, true). They will just hope a baby is born naturally, with no tearing.

They might have heard about caesarean sections and forceps, but many won't know much about them – why they're done, how often they're done, how they're done. They will just hope these won't be done to them.

I suspect that many expectant mothers stumble into labour knowing far less than they may wish to about a big day that could end with a vaginal birth, a forceps or vacuum birth, or a caesar. Many will have gathered their sum knowledge of childbirth from a few evenings of birth classes (which are valuable for sure but perhaps cannot hope to cover many facts women may wish to know) possibly coloured by animated accounts from friends with varying birth experiences. It is a scary thought that many will know far more about the unsavoury habits, dreams and desires of their favourite reality TV star than what could befall them in the birth suite.

And so, I offer this book so that expectant mums can step into the birth day empowered by knowledge. Because knowledge can remove fear. Removing fear can make childbirth more rewarding. And a rewarding childbirth is a perfect springboard to motherhood.

Modern women making their mark in this frenetic world are busy people. Their time is precious and should be respected. And let's face it, planning a wedding is way more fun than boning up on the finer points of childbirth. Therefore, I have tried to keep this book short; it's an easy read that can be digested with focused reading in lieu of a few evenings of Netflix. And perhaps a thumb-through closer to the big day.

I have also written this for birth partners and the privileged few invited to support someone giving birth: mums, dads, sisters, friends and so on. This book will help them learn about what might happen and why they play such a valuable role merely by being there.

What may set this book apart from the remarkably few on the topic of birth (there are loads more suggesting ingenious ways to declutter, or how to say no) is that I am completely neutral. I write with no staunch philosophy on how women should approach labour. I simply aim to offer the facts on modern, safe obstetrics care that has evolved and been refined over centuries. I am just as delighted whether women decide to give acupuncture a shot, opt for hypnobirthing or other meditation techniques to manage pain during labour, content to simply play it by ear on the big day, wish to avoid an epidural, red-hot keen for an epidural to be slotted in as early as possible, or have even made their own informed decision to birth via a planned caesarean section. I hope this book can help them with all those decisions.

Alice's two birth experiences

Let's begin by reflecting on two very different birth experiences.

Vignette 1

Arms enveloping her precious newborn, Alice was amazed how smoothly it went – a view affirmed by her midwife Jane, who agreed it was quite the dream birth. Sure, the pains of labour were no fun, but Alice had weathered them with the support of Jack, Jane, the soothing tones of Enya and a purple bouncy ball. After arriving at the birth suite just after eight, she'd had a pleasingly rapid labour and reached full cervical dilation by mid-morning. Just three robust pushes and baby Lucinda emerged. No tearing. The placenta slid out quietly, almost unnoticed. A beam of glorious sunlight shot forth through the window, a golden beam of radiant warmth bathing mother and cooing newborn.

Vignette 2

The day started well. Alice arrived at the birth suite by sunrise. Greeted with a smile from Jane the midwife, her labour was in full flight by mid-morning. But as labour stretched into the afternoon progression had stopped, though the excruciating pains persisted. By late afternoon Alice, already exhausted, was informed that her cervix had remained stubbornly unchanged at 5 centimetres dilatation. Passage of the baby down the birth canal had stopped dead halfway to full cervical dilation. She was told she had probably stopped dilating because the baby was in a posterior position – baby's back lined up directly with hers and the baby faced upwards towards the ceiling. Apparently, this slows labour. A drip was now needed to strengthen the contractions. It was going to be a long birth.

With the drip ramping up the contractions (and the pain), by late evening Alice slowly edged to full dilatation. She then pushed for two hours, an ordeal that was way harder than she had imagined. Dripping with sweat, exhausted to the bone and now running a fever, she was crestfallen that no baby had appeared. Labour remained upon Alice.

Things then became more urgent. During all the pushing the baby's heart rate sped up. The continuous fetal heart rate monitor that had been on all afternoon had noticeably quickened in pace; it was now tapping at a seemingly improbable 180 beats per minute. Without knowing what it all meant, the noisy uptick in the speed of the fetal heart struck terror in Alice.

Night – day – night. Trapped in a long unrelenting labour. How was the baby going to get out? Will it ever? A doctor then drew up a chair beside Alice. She gathered a tense smile and murmured softly, 'The baby is still facing the wrong way. It's getting distressed. We need to chat…'

You don't need to have given birth before to realise that if given the choice, we'd all run with the first scenario. I would like to offer a few thoughts as we mull over these birth experiences.

First, I am happy to say that a vaginal birth is more likely than a labour that runs aground. Most vaginal births do not flow quite as smoothly as Alice's 'made for TV' birth in the first vignette (though I have indeed witnessed a few that were pretty close), but most will get there.

However, even for those destined for a vaginal birth I suspect that the experience could be made far more rewarding and less scary if women knew more about it before it happens. A somewhat extreme analogy may be to imagine a young adult emerging for the first time from sheltered tribal life, previously hidden away on a dense jungle island. Still dazzled by the bling of modern technology, they are booked to hop on a commercial long-haul flight (clearly paid for by an opportunistic promoter) but knows nothing about planes. Never seen one before. Now, because they are flying with a reputable airline you and I know that they will safely reach their destination (statistically a far safer journey than the next one, where the sleezy promoter picks the chap up at the airport in his hotted-up red Porsche). But isn't it likely that we could convert a terrifying experience into an enjoyable one if they were told some basic facts before the flight? That turbulence can happen but is usually perfectly safe, variably tasty meals will be served on very small trays, steer clear of grumpy-looking cabin crew, it's best to surrender all armrest real estate to the tattooed beefcake next to them, don't make eye contact with the crew member selling duty free, and anticipate the evils of jetlag.

Similarly, I would imagine women will find the journey of a vaginal birth less scary and more fulfilling if they have a good handle on what *could* happen. Hence, most of this book will be spent walking the reader through 'plan A' – a vaginal birth. I cover how long labour lasts, pain relief options (including the ins and outs of an epidural), why vaginal examinations are done, why we doctors and midwives take such a keen interest in the baby's heart rate patterns during labour, why tearing happens and how it is safely mended, what placentas are for and what is done to keep women safe if they start to bleed heavily after the birth. And, importantly, how to push.

The scenario of an obstructed labour – one that does not progress and needs some medical assistance – is not that uncommon. It happens, I'm afraid. And perhaps more often than you'd might think. It may surprise you that around 30–50 per cent of first-time mothers in Australia need a helping hand to birth their child, either by forceps, ventouse (or vacuum – I use these terms interchangeably in this book) or a caesarean section.

This leads me to my second thought. For women going into labour, the way a baby will be ultimately birthed is uncertain right up until the end. When you think about it, it's amazing that, even in this day and age, when expectant mothers step into the birth suite no-one can safely predict whether she will wind up with a natural birth, forceps or a birth by caesarean section. Often, we will only find out within the last hour before birth itself. This is particularly true for first-time mums. We can guess with more confidence that a second-time mum who had a prior vaginal birth is very likely to do it again. Therefore, it may be worth knowing about all the paths to birth before the big day because no-one knows which will happen for the birth that you will be involved in.

My last thought concerns time. Once a clinical decision is made to proceed with forceps or a caesar, events move swiftly. A common reason why we need to act with haste is that we may be concerned that the baby is coping badly with the stress of labour; he is suffering from a poor flow of oxygen and at risk.

This makes things time critical. Most forceps or vacuum births are completed within half an hour of the decision that one is needed, and caesars are done within an hour or two.

This presents a difficult practical dilemma: once a medical decision has been made to undertake a forceps or a caesar birth, there is a terribly short window of time for the clinical team to tell women all about the procedure and why we recommend it. And often little to no time for women to digest it all. This is not ideal.

What's worse is that when we are trying to feed quite a volume of important information to women within the shortest possible time, they are often in the midst of a brutally long labour. They are simply exhausted and aren't in the best state to intellectually engage with a barrage of facts lobbed at them.

There is no easy solution. Having managed this stuff in birth suites for some 20 years now, I reasoned that one answer is to offer information in a book that expectant women (and her nominated support team for the big day) can absorb at their leisure, well ahead of birth. By acquiring knowledge in advance, women will be in a better position to offer true informed consent if their labours stray off the path of a vaginal exit for baby. The procedures recommended may become far less scary if women knew a lot about them beforehand.

The layout of my book is straightforward. Chapter 1 is an overview of labour and childbirth and the whole process leading up to the big moment. We then take a closer look at pain relief options in Chapter 2. Chapter 3 covers ways labour can begin – naturally or with some prompting. Chapters 4, 5 and 6 step through the three stages of labour. Finally, we turn our minds to the plan Bs of childbirth: assistance using forceps or ventouse (vacuum), and caesarean sections (see Chapters 7 and 8).

I address you, the reader, throughout the book, but because the reader may not always be someone who is expecting, I refer to the person giving birth in the third person – 'mum' rather than 'you'. Note that I've used 'mum' – so I didn't have to use 'the mother' or 'the woman' all the time; and that's how we refer to them in the biz – 'mums'. I have used the pronouns she/her for the birthing parent. I have mainly referred to the birthing partner as exactly that (or used gender neutral terms), but on occasion refer to them as he/him, spouse or dad. I realise these descriptions may not represent all the wonderful faces of modern parenting and I apologise if the text does not always suit the pronoun (or relationship status) that you identify with.

Sometimes, rather than using the clunky 'his/her', I simply refer to the baby as 'him' or 'her'; for example, 'the baby switches to her own lungs to draw breath' or 'for additional clues as to which direction bubby is facing, we can also try to feel where his ears are'. When I talk about 'we' I usually mean the clinical team in the birth suite; for example, 'this is how we induce labour'; but other times 'we' means you, dear reader, and me as we travel on this marvellous journey together.

My singular aim for this book is to demystify the safe, modern care of labour and childbirth so that potentially frightening birth experiences are replaced by rewarding events that become cherished lifelong memories. Let's begin…

Chapter 1

A day to remember: the journey of labour and childbirth

In this era of a stupidly expansive range of brain-rotting movies that can be instantaneously streamed at a tap of a button, I often dig around the internet to choose one worth watching. A spot of systematic, methodological market research. First, I scroll about the Netflix site eyeballing the bamboozling array of movies I can pick. I might do a few specific searches just to be sure (yet again) that the blockbusters I actually wish to view are still not available on Netflix, although I will always be reassured there are 20 on offer that are similar (according to Netflix anyway, though I imagine they will be more B-grade and far less blockbustery).

After half an hour of indecision, I shortlist a few: an intellectually driven choice based on high quality information – the title alone and whether the movie poster the size of a postage stamp catches my eye above the many other tempting offerings tiled around it.

To make a final choice among my shortlist I turn to that most reputable source of erudition, the knowledge fountain of pure truth. Wikipedia. There, I hunt for snippets on each movie with keen regard, facts that in all probability have no relevance as to how much I will end up enjoying it. The Wikipedia entry provides the Rotten Tomatoes score and I am turned off if it is lower than 35 per cent. (Unless the film includes Jason Statham, an underrated classical actor who never fails to dispatch baddies in a most satisfying 'butt-kicking' manner, whether it is a menacing gangster or a gigantic prehistoric megalodon shark who is a little perplexed why it finds itself paddling about crowded beaches of modern-day China, but is nevertheless feeling peckish.) Finally, I do a little maths, deducting the cost to make the film from box office earnings to see whether it was a hit or a flop.

But here is the thing. I am always super careful to avoid the plot summary that lurks on the same Wikipedia webpage. If I accidentally read the plot twist, I bin the movie (hey, there are gazillions more to choose from).

Well, this is what this chapter is: the plot summary of the book. The 'beware, spoilers ahead' movie review. Why would I add something like this when I am so careful to avoid spoilers myself? The difference is that this book is factual, and I am trying to convey information to busy readers in the most efficient way possible. And I think it is easier to learn something if you are first offered a skeleton of the topic. And that's what this chapter aims to be. In subsequent chapters, I add flesh to the skeleton with more interesting detail.

So here it is. The plot summary of childbirth.

What's inside the pregnant uterus?

The unborn baby rests neatly folded within the uterus which, in essence, is a big bag of muscle. But what a remarkable one. In the non-pregnant state, the uterus is as small as a Josephine pear delicately perched upside down in the pelvis. When called to action it stretches. And stretches. Ridiculously. Without adding to its complement of existing cells, the bag that is the uterus elongates so magnificently that by the end of pregnancy it obligingly houses a baby of some 3 or 4 kilograms in weight contentedly sloshing about in 500 millilitres of straw-coloured liquid called amniotic fluid, which mainly comes from its bladder (it is a charming thought that we all begin life in utter darkness bathed in our own wee). In addition, the uterus also accommodates the dense, meaty placenta weighing in at around 600 grams. All held in without complaining, seemingly without effort, nice and watertight. A feat I daresay Elastigirl could not hope to match.

The opening of the uterus facing the birth canal is the cervix and it is a major player in childbirth. It is nestled at the lower end of the uterus and sits at the upper end of the vagina, or birth canal. Shaped rather like a mini donut, the hole in the middle of the cervix forms a continuous tunnel from the vagina to the inside space (or 'cavity') of the uterus where the unborn baby is housed. On the day of childbirth, the tiny hole in the centre of the cervix gapes to a whopping 10 centimetres, large enough to permit the baby to pass. Within minutes after the placenta is delivered the cervix closes rapidly. All in all, the uterus is one capable, stretchy organ.

The placenta is a fleshy disc with a remarkably similar diameter to a small pizza from Dominos, though a fair bit thicker. You may disapprove of my comparison as distasteful, but in fact 'placenta' and 'pizza' are both derived from the word 'cake'. One side - the 'maternal side' - is firmly embedded in the inner lining of the uterine cavity. It's the surface that sucks up nutrients and oxygen from mum's blood.

Emerging from the centre on the other side - the fetal side of the placenta - is the umbilical cord. Some fifty centimetres in length, it floats about in the amniotic fluid as coiled loops. The other end of the cord ends at the belly button of the unborn baby, feeding the fetal blood vessels within the cord itself into the baby where they seamlessly join the fetal circulation. In fact, this is exactly what belly buttons are for. I am fairly sure their original purpose was not to be a convenient nub of flesh that is pierced with decorative sharp metal objects. Or to trap fluff.

Extending outwards as continuous sheets from the edges of the placenta and draping the walls of the uterine cavity like a carpet are the placental membranes. 'They', for there are two layers, keep things watertight by holding in all the amniotic fluid in the uterus with the developing baby floating within. If the placental membranes spring a leak then amniotic fluid will drip (or gush) out of the vagina and this is what's widely known as 'the waters breaking'.

The placenta ain't the loveliest to behold. The maternal side looks like chunks of lumpy exposed flesh; dark brown in hue with a shiny wet gleam. In fact it doesn't just look like that – it is that. Coursing along the surface of the fetal side of the placenta are a dense tangle of freaky looking chubby blood vessels, ones that Hollywood might decorate nasty alien beings with malicious intent. Post birth, the placenta can emerge quite bloodied. And a little whiffy too. At times it can have a green tinge. Given its disagreeable appearance it's perhaps not surprising that the poor placenta often fails to feature in even a single photo among daddy's expansive happy snaps capturing the joyous day of childbirth. I just can't quite believe some are moved to turn them into capsules and swallow them.

While not the prettiest to look at the placenta is incredibly beautiful in what it does. During the long months of pregnancy, it is the life support system of the developing human. The placenta continuously sips oxygen and nutrients from mum's blood that runs along the border of the placenta itself and concentrates these goodies in the fetal blood, which is then gathered into major blood vessels that lead to the umbilical cord. The fetal blood is then transported from the placenta through the umbilical cord (via the belly button) into the fetal circulation.

In turn the placenta facilitates the disposal of waste products such as carbon dioxide, palming it off from the fetal circulation to the mothers', to be harmlessly washed away. The placenta is the reason why unborn babies can thrive submerged in amniotic fluid – they are not using their lungs to inhale oxygen. Us humans of now, and of generations past only exist – only have ever existed - because there was once a placenta sustaining us. Our life support system. A remarkable organ. If we ponder what a loyal, useful, benevolent and selfless structure it is, it's pretty sad we do not regard it with the respect it deserves. Instead, after birth we casually toss it into a yellow bag, earmarked for obliteration by extreme temperature incineration.

The length of pregnancy and labour

The 'expected date of birth' or the 'due date' is traditionally calculated as precisely 40 completed weeks from the first day of the last menstrual period. It can also be determined by an ultrasound performed during the first trimester of pregnancy, as early as six to thirteen weeks. The ultrasound method is simple. We measure the length of the fetus – called the embryo at this early stage – and look up a reference chart. For example, an embryo measuring 15 millimetres in length (the 'crown-rump' length) will be seven weeks, plus six days old on the day of the scan. Then, from the date of the ultrasound we derive the expected date of birth by adding 32 weeks and a day (arriving at exactly 40 weeks and zero days).

Dating a pregnancy by ultrasound is more accurate than calculating it based on period dates because natural variations in the length of menstrual cycles between women introduces uncertainty: dating according to period dates assumes an egg is released precisely 14 days after the first day of the last period, which is not always true. Also, many women are simply unsure when their last period began.

The expected date of delivery, or 40 weeks gestation, is an arbitrary line in the sand – very few women will birth on that exact day. Pregnant women become more and more likely to go into natural (or 'spontaneous') labour as they edge closer to 40 weeks gestation.

Most babies are born just before 40 weeks gestation; however, some will overshoot this auspicious day by a week or so. This can stress expectant women who are already on high alert, have their bags all packed (and for many, repeatedly repacked) and dismayed to find themselves still pregnant. They may become unsettled by a new numbering system, where counting towards 40 weeks abruptly pivots to counting upwards. One day over. Two days over. Tomorrow it'll be three … is something wrong? Saintly patience is needed for women who glide past their due date and they should be reassured that many pregnancies do this. If labour hasn't arrived by around 41 weeks gestation, women will be offered an induction of labour within the next week or so, as it can become too risky for babies to remain in the womb beyond 42 weeks of pregnancy. The reason is that by this time, many placentas are past their prime and the risk of stillbirth increases sharply. Chapter 3 talks more about spontaneous labour and how we give things a move along if needed.

Labour lasts around eight hours for a first-time mother and is usually a fair bit shorter for those who have birthed before. However, there is dramatic variation in how long labour can last. Some first-time mothers are blessed with a speedy birth – aka Alice, vignette one (whom we met in the introduction). But for those who do go quickly they should consider themselves warned that they risk becoming the focus of envy at future dinner parties if conversations dare stray into the fraught territory of personal childbirth experiences (where for the rest of the dinner they risk getting a cold shoulder from mums who endured an epic labour, aka Alice, vignette two).

Sadly, the eight hours only counts the period of 'active labour'; where strong, painful contractions are in full flight. It does not include the many hours of 'passive labour', which is the slow build-up of uterine contractions. The passive stage can also be quick or hang about for days – a tiresome situation we call 'spurious labour'.

Labour comes in three stages imaginatively termed the first, second and third (see Chapters 4, 5 and 6 respectively). The first stage starts with the arrival of active contractions and cervix dilatation and ends when the cervix is fully open, or 'fully dilated' (10 centimetres open). Most of the time spent in labour is during the first stage. And I am afraid it can get rather uncomfy. The second stage is declared at full cervical dilatation and is at an end with the arrival of baby. It lasts around one to three hours and includes the infamous period of pushing. Again, it can be far shorter, even a matter of minutes for some really lucky ones. The third and final stage starts from the birth of baby and ends when the placenta has slid out. This is usually done and dusted within 10–15 minutes, and should last no longer than an hour.

Contractions, getting into labour and the first stage

One day, the uterus will start contracting. With each contraction the muscle fibres in the uterus shorten in unison and the uterus squeezes tight, then relaxes as the contraction falls away. Muscle fibres make up the upper and middle sections of the uterus whereas the lower third, called the 'lower segment', is made up of fibrous tissue that doesn't contract. Successive waves of muscle contractions squeeze the upper two thirds of the uterus, which edges the baby down slowly but inexorably (hopefully) through the birth canal. It is a little like squeezing the top of a plastic tomato sauce bottle to add a delicious condiment to a steamy hot dog. But with the minor difference that it can take eight hours of repetitive squeezing before anything emerges (at which time the hot dog might be less steamy).

What the uterus does really is remarkable. In a process that remains cloaked in mystery, the uterus somehow coordinates the simultaneous shortening (or contraction) of millions upon millions of single muscle fibres with a regularity that is impressively precise. How do they all know to contract then relax at the same time? (Are they telepathic?) Furthermore, this amazing structure lies dormant for decades with the annoying need for tampons being the only evidence of its existence. While pregnant, the uterus somehow knows to resist contracting for months on end despite being stretched terrifically, springs into frenetic action on that one special day of childbirth, then shrinks down to its former pear-like dimensions to resume quiet living.

In the beginning, the early contractions are not painful. It feels as though the uterus becomes tight as if it is scrunching into a ball, then relaxes again. This pain can be distinguished from ligament pain (a terribly common and pesky symptom of pregnancy) by the fact that it is centred on the uterus rather than lower down in the pelvis, they last around 10–15 seconds, and recur at roughly 10–15 minutely intervals. With time they gradually increase in frequency, strength and intensity. This is the above mentioned 'passive stage' of labour, and women are often encouraged to stay at home as it can last a while.

Eventually this build-up spills into active labour, where there may be three or more decent contractions within each successive 10-minute 'block' of time. Most birth suites will invite women in when they are feeling two decent contractions (each lasting around 30 seconds or so) within every 10-minute block and this provides a pretty safe margin; it is very rare that women will not make it to the birth suite in time.

During active labour each contraction lasts around 60–90 seconds. There will be three to four of these within every 10-minute block of time. And I'm afraid the pain can be pretty intense. We staff in the birth suite will not be convinced that women are in active labour if they are able to comfortably chat during contractions. Thankfully, there is complete respite from pain between contractions and they magically cease the moment baby is born.

At the beginning of active labour, the cervix is usually 2–3 centimetres open, or dilated. It first needs to dilate to 10 centimetres, or full dilatation. Once fully dilated, the second stage commences and the mum-to-be can proceed with pushing out her little angel. So, in essence, the first stage is all about waiting for full cervical dilatation.

We assess the degree of cervical dilatation by performing regular vaginal (or internal) examinations during labour, roughly four hours apart. At full dilatation no cervix can be felt by the gloved examiner, only the baby's head filling the pelvis.

The vaginal examination can also determine which way the baby is facing. Ideally, the unborn baby should be facing down towards the ground (or towards mum's back), that is, orientated so her mouth is closer to mum's anus, the eyes closer to mum's pubic bone (the top of her head gliding just under the bone). This is the 'occipital anterior' position, and it is optimal because this position naturally makes the baby flex (or bend) her neck and tuck her chin onto her chest. In fact, ideally the neck is so flexed that the leading edge of the baby coming through the birth canal is the top and back of her head, not the eyes. This creates the smallest possible head diameter to squeeze through the vaginal opening. It is possible to give birth vaginally if the baby is coming out in different positions, such as the 'occipital posterior position' (orientated so that the eyes are closer to the anus and the mouth closer to mum's pubic bone) but this usually a fair bit more involved.

You can imagine that women in the first stage of active labour need to deal with waves of painful contractions which roll on for many plodding hours. It can be pretty taxing stuff. The good news is that there will be a dedicated team that will take great care of her. Central to the team will be a caring midwife, a highly trained birth attendant. They will be a really comforting presence providing comfort, reassurance and 'on the spot' expertise as events unfold.

Also part of the team keeping mum and baby safe will be one of us, an obstetrician. To become a specialist obstetrician we first train as medical doctors, then face the rigours (some might say the horrors) of four to six years of specialist obstetrics training so that we can call ourselves experts in the care of pregnant women. We work shoulder to shoulder with midwives as an integrated team. The obstetrician provides overall supervision, takes overall responsibility and is on tap to render assistance for labours that aren't travelling smoothly. We are the ones trained to perform caesarean sections ('caesars'), forceps or vacuums if they are needed and we take charge if complications surface. But we are not just there for the difficult stuff. We also enjoy being involved in normal vaginal births.

Sometimes, the doctor is a highly skilled general practitioner (or a primary care physician) who has a special interest in caring for women while they birth. Depending on their level of training they may also have the skills to perform vacuums or caesars should they be needed.

We mustn't forget that spouses or birth partners form a vital part of the support crew. They play a crucial role providing a bedrock of emotional support. If you are one, you will probably find the person you are supporting will not be in the mood for small talk during labour: they just want the nurturing attention of their hand-picked support team. A well-timed hug can be of inestimable comfort. And if you are a support person bear in mind that while in the birth suite it's not the time to catch up on Facebook or emails. Not a furtive glance; not a quick Instagram post. Don't tweet updates. It really isn't a good look when we see the birth partner constantly distracted by their phone or distracted by anything. And we see it. I recall one support partner who stepped out of the birthing room, snuck off to the staff tearoom and rifled through the staff's belongings, pinching purses. Not cool.

Other things can be tried to set the mood. Fake candles with a soft, mesmerising flicker. Or real ones if the birth suite permits them. Dimmed lights. And music – Kenny G and Enya once dominated the aural ambience of birth suites during the late 1990s but are now (mercifully) replaced by all manner of music styles streamed via Spotify. Hard rock is actually not all that infrequent. But many labouring women do not bother with such frills and do just fine.

Options for pain relief

There are different things labouring women can try out to cope with the pains that occur with contractions; plenty of courses, books and blogs teach meditative techniques (body-mind-uterus), many with a focus on breathing. Women can pace about, stand and sway, lightly bounce on a large sturdy birth ball; some are content to simply lie in bed, semi-upright or even lying on their backs (though with a slight tilt to the left, made possible by strategically positioned pillows). Some find a soak in the bath or the trickle of a warm shower soothing (as we shall find out later, there is some science to this). A shoulder massage can be useful, but it only seems to work if willingly offered by the tender hands of a loving partner. Heat packs across the lower back can also provide relief.

There are a quite a few other pain relief options. Women can breathe in nitrous oxide during the contraction, colloquially known as 'laughing gas'. Another alternative is a 'TENS' machine, the short form of the rather ostentatious 'Trans-cutaneous electrical nerve stimulation'. At the push of a button the TENS machine relays electrical pulses to small pads dotted along the lower back. The TENS machine triggers the sensation of touch which jostle for the brain's attention, competing with electrical impulses from the uterus propagating the sensation of pain. The net effect is that the signal from the TENS machine may help dull the pain. Other things that can be tried include aromatherapy, acupuncture (by prior arrangement with an acupuncturist) and water injections into the back. The biological basis underpinning some of these approaches is a little controversial, but they are all very safe. And if a labouring woman finds any to be helpful then I enthusiastically approve of them.

A stronger pain relief option is an injection of an opiate drug, such as morphine (some units may use pethidine). These can decrease the intensity of the pain for a few hours. However, opiates can make you spewy, so we commonly administer anti-vomiting medications at the same time. The slight concern with opiate injections is that if birth happens within two to three hours after the injection, bubby might emerge a little dozy and require a little breathing support from a paediatric team soon after birth until the effects wear off. But if it happens, it's usually short lived and harmless.

The options mentioned so far can take the edge off the pain but fall short of removing the pain. However, they may be sufficient for many, especially those who are blessed with speedy births. The only way to completely remove the pain is to have an epidural. When running well it is dramatically effective.

The epidural is a very fine tube introduced via a needle into the lower back. And I mean really fine, just a millimetre in thickness. The introducer needle is removed after the epidural catheter (aka the super thin tube) is in place, and only the tube is left in the back. When slotted in, there is no big filthy needle left dangling out of the back.

One end of the epidural catheter rests delicately in one of the spaces within the lower back near the spine (but well clear from the important knot of nerves that form the spinal cord itself). The other end of the tube emerges through a microscopic hole in the back, runs up along the skin of the back towards the shoulder and ends attached to a drug infusion pump suspended in mid-air on a pole beside the bed. This allows the continuous infusion of precise doses of local anaesthetic agents that drip into the back, blocking nerves that sense pain from the uterus.

Often, the pain reducing medications dripped through the epidural catheter cannot be finessed to selectively block pain fibres alone; they can also affect the nerves controlling leg movement. This means women with epidurals running generally cannot reliably stand and may need to lounge in bed until they birth their baby. Also, those with an epidural cannot feel when they need to pee so a urinary catheter is slotted in via the urethra (the wee hole) to keep the bladder empty. Otherwise, the bladder could fill up and become overly stretched and damaged.

Within hours of birth the epidural catheter is whipped out, leg control will quickly return, and a welcome shower can soon follow.

Epidurals have a bad rep

For some reason, a glaring spotlight is firmly fixed on the epidural as a focal point of political exchange, heated discussion and resolute social opinion that is broadcast freely (and loudly) whether solicited or not. Friends may enquire with unabashed directness, 'Are you going to try without an epidural?' I recently heard a complete stranger ask a new mother, 'Did you *need* an epidural?' A frenemy may announce with pride that they toughed it out without one, which can seem like a subtle challenge to expectant mums within earshot. To add to the quagmire, some vocal 'experts' resolutely declare that the epidural is the very invention of the devil; a weapon of disempowerment that triggers a 'cascade of interventions', thrusting the hapless victim into a treacherous, swirling whirlpool of increasingly dangerous and wholly avoidable medical procedures (as I will discuss in the next chapter, this is untrue).

I think it is a terrible shame that the epidural has become so politicised. It is just one pain relief option, no more, no less (albeit a very effective one). It is very safe and has legions of satisfied customers but also carries some small risks. Some will opt for it and others won't.

I am a fan of the epidural simply because it is just so effective at taking the pain away. Even though I have loitered about in various birth suites across two decades (hey, I am not that ancient) I still hate seeing people languishing in pain who do not wish to be, looking terribly despondent and deflated. In such cases the epidural can not only dispatch with the pain but boost the mood. This isn't to say for a minute that everyone should have one. In the next chapter, I dig deeper into the pros and cons of an epidural. For now, suffice it to say that the decision whether to have one surely rests with the labouring woman. Her choice should not merely be 'accepted' but be unjudged, and enthusiastically supported. Her decision-making should not be burdened by what others might think of it, and of them.

By now I hope you have acquired a flavour of the first stage of labour: roughly how long it lasts, how we determine progress (by performing regular vaginal examinations), and pain relief options. And I hope you are reassured that there will be the comforting presence of a skilled midwife constantly by the side of someone who is labouring, and that mum may also be cared for by skilled obstetricians (or general practitioners). With some imagination you may even manage to conjure up an image of the scene in the birth suite. But before we arrive at the second stage of labour, let's turn to the other important player who is deeply invested in the big day going right, though they aren't aware of it at the time (in fact, they are aware of very little of anything): the unborn baby.

Keeping the baby safe during labour

You may have heard that the clinical team closely monitors the baby's heart rate during labour and wondered why. The reason is that labour can be a risky time for unborn babies and monitoring the fetal heart rate patterns points us to those in strife because they aren't getting the oxygen they need.

With their lungs lying dormant before birth, unborn babies depend on their placentas as their sole source of oxygen. The placenta itself receives a constant flow of fresh oxygen from mum's blood vessels and these reach the placenta after weaving through a lattice of muscle that forms the wall of the uterus. When the uterus squeezes into a tight ball during contractions the maternal blood vessels running within are squished. Happily, the baby gets to breathe between contractions because the uterine muscles relax, and the squeeze on the blood vessels ease. However, the net effect is that as labour progresses the total amount of oxygen delivered from mother to unborn baby reduces as the hours tick by.

During labour it's a bit like the baby is running a marathon. It's a test of endurance. Most cope just fine and are only a little puffed by the end of the race. A small number may have struggled throughout the run and reach the finish line profoundly exhausted. They may stagger through the red ribbon at the finish line (in this analogy, this is birth itself) and collapse into the attentive arms of first aid officers on standby (aka the paediatric team attending birth, which I talk more about later). Although bone-weary, these babies will be just fine because their marathon is at an end. With the race finished they can rest and suck in all the oxygen they need. Importantly, they have reached the care of the first aid officers who have a range of options to revive them back to health.

But a yet smaller number may fail entirely to cope with the run midway. They simply cannot summon the energy to reach the finishing line. The situation is more grave for unborn babies who do not have the option to simply stop running; they find themselves trapped in a hostile environment of stiflingly low oxygen well before full cervical dilation. And still a long distance from being safely born. Without access to a speedy caesarean section some babies in this hapless quandary won't make it out of the uterus alive. Others might just escape alive but tumble out silent with a thready pulse, and manage to just survive with a prolonged period of intensive resuscitation efforts. But this is not a flash way to begin life – such babies have a risk of being permanently scarred with serious disability from brain tissue damage caused by an overly long period of very low oxygen while stuck in the womb.

How do we clinicians sift out the few babies in peril that need us to intervene with a lifesaving caesarean section among the many others coping just fine with labour? If there was some form of technology that could accurately tell us the precise, minute-by-minute oxygen levels in the unborn fetus during labour we'd use it. But we don't.

However, researchers some six decades ago discovered specific heart rate patterns that appear in unborn babies who are suffocating from low oxygen levels. This led to the rapid clinical adoption of fetal heart rate monitoring, called the 'cardiotocograph' (known widely as the 'CTG'). The CTG monitors fetal heart rate patterns continuously, sort of like an electrocardiogram (or ECG) of the baby (though it's not quite the same thing). The appearance of specific fetal heart rate patterns can raise suspicions there may be dangerous fetal distress caused by low oxygenation. Seeing these will prompt the clinical team to have a careful think about whether it is necessary to fast-track birth to keep baby safe. Occasionally we need to act super swiftly if really ominous fetal heart rate patterns appear.

During the first stage of labour (where the cervix has not reached full dilatation) the only way to expedite birth is by caesarean section. In the second stage, the choices to expedite birth are a caesar or an instrumental birth, which will either be a forceps or vacuum birth. The choice between a caesar or an instrumental birth is made depending on how low the baby has descended down the birth canal and the direction it's facing. Caesars, forceps and vacuums will be touched on later in this chapter, then covered in quite some detail towards the end of this (riveting) book.

Hence, the last jigsaw piece you may wish to add to the imagery of the birth suite in your mind's eye is that we will be monitoring the fetal heart rate. If the pregnancy is considered low risk then the midwife will intermittently use the hand-held Doppler device to listen to the fetal heart – the same device used at antenatal visits (the portable machine which makes the fetal heartbeat sound like horses galloping). If there are any underlying concerns with the pregnancy or the hand-held Doppler device raises suspicion that a concerning heart rate pattern may be present, then we switch over to the CTG to continuously monitor fetal heart rate patterns. Unlike the hand-held Doppler, the CTG provides a constant readout and conveys more detailed information. Once the CTG is applied, the baby's heart rate patterns are monitored through labour, right up until bub is safely born and clear of harm's way.

The second stage of labour

After many uncomfortable hours and resolute determination on the part of the brave mum-to-be, the midwife or obstetrician performs a vaginal examination and declares the cervix to be fully dilated. Yippee. We have arrived at the second stage.

The second stage lasts roughly one to two hours. Like the first stage, timelines can vary wildly. It can be mercifully short, especially for second-time mums, and even a matter of minutes for those who have had many vaginal births before. But for some unlucky ones, it can drag on beyond two hours. We do not really like the second stage stretching beyond three hours as the risks to baby (and even to mum) start to lift.

Like the first stage, the second is divided into 'passive' and 'active' stages. The passive stage is an arbitrary period of time when we encourage women not to push. This is to allow the baby to descend down the birth canal as low as possible under the steam of further uterine contractions before we ask mum to exert herself. The active stage begins when the 'almost mum' starts her almighty pushes. The purpose of the passive stage – waiting for a while before pushing – is to move the starting line closer to the finish, so as to shorten the length of the run (aka the length of time that is spent pushing, or the 'active' second stage).

During the active stage women are encouraged to push during uterine contractions and rest during the minute or so between them. Pushing is a pretty strenuous workout and should be focused on the same spot to ease out a poo, but with far greater explosive force than what is typically required for number twos (unless there is zero fibre intake). A common technique is to fill the lungs by a little more than half before a sustained push – as hard as possible – that lasts for an effortful 10–15 seconds. A push with as much strength that the mum-to-be can possibly muster. We are talking beetroot red face, determined grimace, strands of saliva dancing about tensed lips, taut neck veins. A burger with the lot.

No air should escape from the mouth during a push as it wastes precious energy. At the end of each push the mum should snatch her breath as quickly as possible – a super speedy exhale and inhale – then immediately commence the next sustained push. All up, for every minute-long uterine contraction there should optimally be a set of three (or four) consecutive pushes where each lasts for about 10–15 seconds, with only the briefest microsecond snatch of breath between them.

The mum-to-be should make full use of the respite between contractions and catch her breath (literally and emotionally) because the next contraction will descend again upon her in a minute or two's time and the next cycle of pushing begins.

Women will often push lying semi upright in bed, but they can push in different positions. They most certainly do not need to be in bed. They can stand, squat or be positioned on 'all fours', with knees and arms on the ground and back in the air (just how we'd imitate a cat to our young kids when clowning about at home, though earnest pushing replaces pretend meow'ing). The experienced midwife can work with the mum to try out different positions.

During all this pushing the support crew around the mum should be her devoted cheer squad, providing moral support that is steadfast and unwavering. Pushing can continue for even an hour or two and lifting the spirits with constant encouragement is supremely important.

Once the baby's head has finally edged down to the opening of the vagina things usually progress a little quicker. The point at which the baby's head is tenting open the vaginal opening and can be directly seen is called 'crowning'. Once this happens birth is tantalisingly close. If an epidural is not on board, this stretch of the vaginal opening causes an unpleasant feeling of intense burning on mum's skin. Happily, the duration is mercifully short: crowning usually lasts around 10–15 minutes and once the baby is out the scorching sensation dissipates.

When the head is born it usually pops out facing downwards toward the floor (mouth closer to mum's anus and eyes closer to her pubic bone). At this point the body is not yet born, it's just the head poking out. The midwife or obstetrician will gently insert a gloved finger to check whether the umbilical cord is looped around the neck of the baby. If so, it's gently loosened and eased out. The head then swivels 90 degrees and the baby ends up facing sideways towards one of mum's thighs. On the next push the shoulders are born, closely followed by the body and legs which all slip out in one smooth slide.

The second stage of labour is an event long remembered by women who have experienced it, as well as her chosen support crew. Although exhausting, it has the satisfying finale of a crying adorable bundle – a warm, wet, slippery new addition to the family plonked onto mum's tummy and into her longing embrace. A cuddle that had been dreamed about for months, possibly years.

The third – and final – stage of labour

Happy times. Baby is out. The horrid painful contractions have shuddered to a halt (good riddance). The terrible burning at the vaginal opening has already started to settle (good riddance to that too). The first strands of an enduring unconditional bond of love between mother and baby are already fast forming. The relieved partner, also exhausted, is darting about the bed, creating happy snaps to capture the precious moment. Gazing at the cooing newborn's face, the parents are already muttering through a shortlist of names to see which best matches junior. And we are in that beautiful zone of pre-social media innocence, an all too brief moment of untainted purity where the birth has still yet to become 'Facebook official'.

However, a few tidying-up things need attending to before the process of childbirth is at an end.

First, we need to deliver the placenta. It usually follows within 10–15 minutes after the baby; however, occasionally it'll be longer. A big, sustained uterine contraction following birth itself shears the placenta off the wall of the uterus where it had been embedded for months. Though detached and floating free, it will still be sitting inside the womb. To coax it out, the midwife or obstetrician places a hand across mum's lower abdomen (to feel where the uterus is) and gently pulls on the umbilical cord with the other hand. Mum doesn't need to push. In fact, often mum hardly notices this is all happening until the placenta plops out.

Occasionally, we encounter a stubborn placenta that refuses to let go of the uterus well after the baby has arrived. A procedure, called a manual removal of placenta, is needed to remove such a nuisance house guest overstaying its welcome. Annoyingly, it is a short trip to theatre where the obstetrician dons a long glove, reaches in via the birth canal into the womb and dislodges the placenta by hand (like a weird version of a forced eviction, I suppose). Sounds yuck but it is a minor procedure that is quick, safe and done under the cover of adequate pain relief so it won't be felt. But it is a bit of a bummer to do as we would all much rather leave the new family in peace. Instead, we need to whisk mum away for a quick visit to the operating suite before returning her back to her prized newborn.

Secondly, concerningly heavy bleeding from the vagina can happen soon after the birth, called a 'postpartum haemorrhage'. We expect some bleeding after all births where anything less than an estimated loss of half a litre is considered acceptable. This sounds like an alarming quantity and I agree you wouldn't want this volume of blood pouring out of a freshly picked nose or scratched pimple. Or from your haemorrhoids. But in the setting of childbirth this is the expected amount and new mothers can tolerate such losses just fine.

If we are concerned that the bleeding is unusually brisk and we estimate that losses are totalling over half a litre we take active measures to stem the flow. The most common source of bleeding is from the inner wall of the uterus itself, from the raw surface where the placenta has freshly detached. Blood trickles from this open surface through the birth canal and out the vagina. To deal with this we rapidly administer drugs to contract the uterus really tightly, and to stay contracted. By squishing the uterus into a very tight ball the blood vessels coursing through it are also squished shut, and this arrests most bleeding. The drugs we give are usually highly effective and stop most cases of haemorrhaging.

In fact, they are unsung heroes and over the recent decades have saved an enormous number of lives.

On occasion these medications fail to stop the bleeding and there is a persistent trickle. If we become concerned that the losses are mounting north of a litre and the bleeding still isn't showing signs of abating, we may need to take the new mum to the operating room so we can try other things to stop the flow (we will cover these later in the book). Luckily, this is very uncommon but utterly annoying when it happens.

Lastly, tearing can happen, caused while bub is squeezing through the vaginal opening. And sometimes, while the head is crowning the midwife or obstetrician will make a small cut at the vaginal opening angled sideways, called an episiotomy. The aim of doing this is to decrease the chance of uncontrolled tears appearing that extend towards the anus and damage the anal sphincter, the important ring of muscle that allows us to control our bowels. The episiotomy tries to direct any tearing away from the anus. Episiotomies are commonly done in the United Kingdom, Europe, Australia and many other regions in the world, but far less so in the United States.

Tearing and episiotomies are common, particularly for first-time mothers, and are expertly mended using stitches (that self-dissolve) very soon after the birth by either the obstetrician, midwife or general practitioner. Happily, the region around the vaginal opening has a plentiful blood supply which endows it the nifty skill of being exceptionally good at healing. It is perhaps similar to our spongy fingertips: being plump with blood, they usually heal exceptionally well without scarring after minor kitchen knife mishaps (even though at the time of the flesh wound they bleed like stink and hurt like heck). Also, most tearing or episiotomies are small and easily repaired with excellent prospects that healing will be quick.

Plan B: caesarean sections, forceps and vacuum (or ventouse) births

If all births progressed smoothly then caesars and forceps would not exist. They simply wouldn't be needed. But the labour does not always follow the elegant path laid out by nature.

There are two main reasons why we turn to caesarean sections or instrumental births (forceps or the vacuum) to expedite birth. The first, which we touched on before, is fetal distress, which is when we have suspicions that the baby may be flagging from stiflingly low oxygen levels, gleaned from concerning fetal heart rate patterns appearing on the CTG machine. Things are different after birth: once out, the baby switches to her own lungs to draw breath, removing the perils faced while in the womb.

The second reason we may recommend a caesar or an instrumental birth to deliver the baby is because there has been arrested progress of labour (sometimes called 'failure to progress'). This is where descent of the baby through the birth canal has stalled. It declares itself during the first stage by the fact that the cervix has stopped dilating, where vaginal examinations spaced many hours apart reveal an infuriating lack of progress. Arrested progress of labour can also happen during the second stage after the cervix has reached full dilatation, where the baby fails to emerge after a long, gallant period of pushing (just ask poor Alice in vignette 2 from the Introduction).

A caesarean section is an operation where we deliver the baby through an abdominal incision, bypassing the vagina entirely: 'The sunroof exit' – more on this in Chapter 8. We make a sideways incision low down on the abdomen, approximately level to the upper border of the bikini line (when fully healed, the skin scar often sits below the upper margin of underwear and hidden from view). We then make a horizontal incision on the uterus and deliver the baby through this incision, and out the hole in the abdominal wall. We then sew up all the layers we opened to reach the baby, one by one. Quite a conceptually simple operation really. With good pain management the recovery can be quite quick; mum will feel pretty comfortable the moment she is wheeled out of the operating theatre, be able to move about on the day of the procedure, be happy to head home after a few nights, and be free of all pain relief medications by about three weeks after the operation.

Forceps can only be deployed in the second stage and are used by obstetricians to help pull out the baby. They look like large salad servers that wrap around and grasp the baby's head.

The two 'blades' of the forceps are eased through the vaginal opening and gently slid around the unborn baby's head, one at a time. When applied, the rounded 'spoon' of the forceps blades hug the baby's cheeks. From the top of bubby's head, the other end of the forceps extend out through the vaginal opening and end as handles that the obstetrician grips. Once the two blades of the forceps are safely placed around the baby's head, they neatly join together. With the onset of a contraction the obstetrician assists birth by pulling on the forceps handles. Once we start tugging on the forceps the baby will usually be birthed within three sets of contractions. The idea of forceps may be a tad intimidating; however, they are cleverly designed to wrap snuggly around the baby's head and centuries of use are testament to its safety.

A vacuum or ventouse birth is similar in concept to the forceps – it's just another way to pull out baby. However, it is a suction cup placed on the baby's head rather than an instrument that wraps around it. The ventouse is shaped somewhat like a sink plunger, or that intimidating stick thingy poking out of evil metallic Daleks (that's for the *Dr Who* fans who have never once cleared a sink blockage before). Except that the suction 'cup' at the end is not as big and is shaped more like a thick round disc about 5–7 centimetres across.

Thin tubing attached to the top of the suction cup runs from the baby's head, through the vaginal opening to a handle with a pump. This hand pump creates a negative pressure inside the cup which provides direct suction on the baby's head (similar in concept to those 1980s TV adverts where a moustache-endowed salesman in a tacky brown suit uses a vacuum cleaner to suck a bowling ball clean in the air to demonstrate its raw power). Like the forceps, the obstetrician pulls on the handle during contractions, and it can only be used during the second stage. Once we have started tugging on the ventouse, birth should be anticipated within three sets of contractions.

Sometimes during labour, the CTG suddenly throws up such alarming fetal heart rate patterns that we are forced to act quickly to remove the baby from serious harm. When this situation arises the window of time to provide information and obtain consent to proceed to a caesar or instrumental birth can be brief.

I hope this has been a useful taste of the different medical interventions; in Chapters 7 and 8, I spend quite some time exploring them in more detail – to really demystify them. So, if they are needed with haste for the birth you are involved in, knowing them well and ahead of time will make the experience far less scary.

There you have it – a bird's eye view of childbirth. I suspect after reading this chapter you will already know a great deal more than many others who step into the birth suite. I am also sort of hoping this chapter has proved surprisingly fascinating to you. And has whet your appetite to discover more (yes, I am just like the many other deluded authors who think their book is interesting).

And there is so much more to discover.

In the next chapter, I will launch into pain relief options. By the end of it you will have acquired a really sound understanding of the many options to counter the pain of labour. Following that, we will take a closer look at the astonishing event that is human labour and childbirth, and what we do if the ship sails off course.

So please stick with me.

Recap:
Overview of birth

1. Spontaneous labour becomes more and more likely to kick in as pregnancies edge closer to the expected date of birth, or 40 weeks gestation. Some perfectly healthy pregnancies overshoot the 'expected date of birth' by one or two weeks.

2. Labour is divided into three stages. The first stage can last six to eight hours, it begins when strong contractions set in, and ends when the cervix is fully dilated. The second stage lasts around one to two hours and is when the mum does her almighty pushing. It concludes when the little munchkin is birthed. The third stage ends when the placenta slides out and is typically over within 15 minutes.

3. Labouring women in the birth suite will be cared for by a highly skilled midwife. Doctors are also an important part of the team. During labour women can take on any position they like; they can eat and play with the ambience of the room (BYO music, aromatherapy, dim the lights, pretend candles, lava lamps).

4. During the first and second stages of labour there are frequent uterine contractions. Unfortunately, they are pretty painful. And intense. Happily, there are a range of options to counter the pain – ranging from non-pharmacological (breathing techniques, TENS machine), inhaling nitric oxide to opioid injections (mainly morphine). An epidural is the most effective option that is dramatically effective in removing the pain altogether.

5. There are two main reasons why we recommend an instrumental birth (forceps or ventouse, widely known as 'the vacuum') or a caesarean section. The first is fetal distress – the unborn baby may be in peril because it's not getting the oxygen it needs (we glean the presence of fetal distress by monitoring fetal heart rate patterns). The second reason we recommend an instrumental birth, or a caesarean section is arrested labour (or 'failure to progress'), where the cervix stops dilating during labour or the baby stops descending down the birth canal during the second stage.

6. If we do need to expedite birth, the only option during the first stage of labour is a caesarean section. For those who have reached the second stage of labour, we will either recommend an instrumental birth (if the baby's head is low enough and it's judged safe to attempt one) or a caesarean section.

Caesareans and instrumental births are very safe, although there are some risks. In coming chapters of this book, I cover caesareans, ventouses and forceps in quite a bit of detail.

Chapter 2

A closer look at pain relief options during labour

Some years back the mathematical genius Jordon Ellenberg came up with the Hawking Index. It (roughly) estimates how often books are read to the very end and is calculated from digital data generated from the millions consuming eBooks on their Kindle devices. It is a disconcerting thought that your ebook reading habits are being hoovered from your password-protected device and freely accessed by numerically gifted strangers in distant lands. Or perhaps in this era no-one cares.

The index is named in honour of the great physicist Stephen Hawking who wrote the mighty *A Brief History of Time*. The name is inspired by the fact that of all the ebook sales of the classic penned by Hawking, only 6.6 per cent were actually read cover to cover (what the index cannot tell us is how many of the 6.6 per cent understood it, which I suspect is not many). I am not surprised. The front pages of my own copy were attacked with inspired enthusiasm, but the latter half remains in mint condition to this day.

Even if you turn to easier reads, the number of books that have engaged the reader to the very end remain surprisingly low. *Catching Fire*, the second *Hunger Games* novel, apparently scores 43.4 per cent. And after the embarrassment of purchasing

Fifty Shades of Grey – albeit online and therefore 'anonymous' – only 25.6 per cent got through all 50 shades. Overall, it is very uncommon for books to crack a score over 50 per cent.

Non-fiction books fare far worse. It was a surprise to me that *How to Win Friends and Influence People* scores a paltry 7.7 per cent (presumably those who bought this timeless self-help classic later decided finding friends wasn't so important after all). Hilary Clinton's memoir, *Hard Choices*, scores a preposterously low 1.9 per cent (any future edition might be more correctly titled *Hard Slog*). You need to search far and wide to find a non-fiction book with a Hawking Index that scores above 20 per cent. I note these truths with some alarm, as *The Birth Book* is also non-fiction.

Thus, the Hawking Index is the unlikely reason why I have prioritised a chapter on pain relief early in the book, before our deep dive into labour. Of course, I would love every one of you devoted readers to consume every morsel of my obvious 'page turner' to the very end (perhaps lingering affectionately on the unique barcode that adorns the back cover), but the Hawking Index tells me that despite my elegant prose and self-declared alluring style some may not make it to the end. Therefore, I have chosen to position the chapter on pain relief early on because I reckon it is one of the most important things that women approaching labour should know well. So important that I have slotted it in the book as early as Chapter 2 in the hope that it lands in your pile marked 'Read'.

The reason why knowing pain relief options well is so vital is that pain relief is the one area where women stepping into the birth suite will have a lot of choice. In fact, they will be asked to actively make choices – to select some pain relief options and consciously decline others. And I am worried that too often, these major decisions are based on no information, incomplete information or even misinformation. My suspicions are backed up by Australian research published in 2007 in the journal *Midwifery*, which concluded pregnant women's understanding of pain relief options are often based on anecdotal information. This is perhaps no surprise to those of us at the front line in the birth suite.

So here they are – the various options to counter pain during labour. I do trust that as you consume this chapter you will tuck away useful facts to draw upon on the big day.

Drug-free strategies

Presumably after some heated exchanges among a panel of esteemed global experts the International Association for the Study of Pain (IASP) pronounced this official definition of pain (as it stood in 2019): 'an unpleasant sensory and emotional experience associated with actual or potential tissue damage, or described in terms of such damage'. Okay…

While an undoubtedly comprehensive definition, it's perhaps a wee bit dry. And although noble in its attempt to cover every conceivable type of pain the earnest panel could think of (and I am sure there were many), this final definition seems rather expansive. According to this definition, just vividly imagining the unpleasant emotional experience of a crazed brown bear ravenously gnawing chunks off one's rapidly diminishing thigh might arguably be defined as pain. And I am also pretty sure this official wording wouldn't be the same verbatim definition if you asked mums to define the pain they experienced during labour. Theirs would likely be shorter and contain risqué words such as 'hurt' (conspicuously absent in the official definition). It might even include a sprinkling of four-letter words that would make illustrious senior committee members of the IASP blush.

Before I get into strife with my professorial academic colleagues, I wish to highlight an important aspect of this official definition of pain espoused by the IASP. Pain is not just sensory, but also an emotional experience. This, I do agree with and is worth bearing in mind when women consider their options for pain relief during labour. Women vary widely in their emotional response to active labour. And it is certainly not the case that those who appear to cope less well are somehow less tough. Not at all. It is simply that humans react in their own personal way to pain, perhaps further influenced by their cultural background and life experiences. For instance, someone who appears to be coping poorly with the pains of early labour may have been anxious for weeks leading up to the event, perhaps frightened by stories told by those around them. This constant anxiety could easily have emotionally sensitised them to react strongly once the pains of active labour finally set in.

Countering the emotional response is a likely explanation why many non-drug (or non-pharmacological) options greatly assist many women to cope with the pain of labour. This is a good thing, as the ultimate goal of pain relief during labour is not so much to minimise the 'unpleasant' sensory pain experience (in non-IASP sanctioned terms, how much it hurts) but to improve the overall emotional experience of childbirth.

Therefore, the presence of hand-selected people in the room – partners, friends and family – is an important way to combat adverse emotional responses to pain during labour. The value of familiar voices uttering soothing messages of encouragement cannot be overestimated. Another strategy is to alter the ambience of the room: candles (even pretend ones), familiar music streamed from a portable speaker or a preselected fragrance wafting from an aromatherapy diffuser to sweeten the aroma of the room. And for some lucky women destined for a rapid labour, such as Alice in the first vignette from the Introduction, such comforting measures may be all that's needed.

Some women opt to invite a doula, a professional support person. Women get to know their doulas ahead of time and they will be a familiar face whose role is not to manage labour but offer emotional support. Many are midwifery trained.

Some women choose a model of private obstetrics care (not all countries offer this). Over the many months of pregnancy, the expectant mother gets to know, bond with and trust the person pegged to assist their birth and this can provide great emotional reassurance during birth. Exactly the same applies to inviting a private midwife (or general practitioner) to provide expert care during pregnancy, and to attend the birth.

Other measures to cope with the pain of contractions are to employ techniques that focus on breathing. Whether they work by distraction, are meditative, or both, I am unsure. But some women find these useful and indeed, I have witnessed many women who manage to enter 'the zone' during the trying hours of labour, breathe through each contraction with full focus and serene determination, and get through a fulfilling birth without medications. For those who are interested there are antenatal courses, such as 'calm birthing' or 'hypnobirthing'.

Gate control theory, TENS machines, water injections and acupuncture

In 1965, Ronald Melzack, a Canadian psychologist, and Patrick Wall, an eminent British neuroscientist, proposed the Gate Control Theory of Pain. The concept is pretty simple. Nerve fibres transmitting the sensation of touch from the skin to the brain are separate to thinner ones that relay the (annoying) feeling of pain. The theory holds that both types of nerve fibres jostle to get their respective messages through the same 'transmission cells' that sit around the spinal cord (the transmission cells then relay the message up the spinal cord to the brain). In essence, the nerves that relay the feeling of touch and pain share the same 'gate'.

If only one nerve type is firing, say the pain fibres, then a message of pain is efficiently relayed via the transmission cells (aka the 'gate') to the brain. And we feel it. But if there is also simultaneous firing of the nerve fibres transmitting a message conveying touch, it will block or decrease the strength of the signal transmitting pain because they can't both efficiently pass through the 'gate' (transmission cells) at the same time.

Gate Control Theory can be intentionally exploited by stimulating touch fibres on the skin to block or at least reduce the strength of the signal conveying pain. One common way we all instinctively use Gate Control Theory to manage the 'unpleasant sensory experience' caused by a bee sting is to give the fresh bite a rub on the skin to dull the sharp pain. (The other way we deal with the 'unpleasant emotional experience' is to murder the pollinating aggressor with unhinged brute force).

Gate Control Theory is probably at play for some of the common drug-free strategies to counter the pain of labour, such as bouncing on a birth ball (where the sensation of touch around the pelvis counters the pain), massage, a shower or bath, or heat packs.

The 'transcutaneous electrical nerve stimulation' (TENS) machine was designed to exploit Gate Control Theory of pain. Four pads housing tiny electrodes are stuck along the lower back. Wires from these pads lead to a machine that pulses electrical signals to stimulate the nerve fibres conveying light touch. The electrical signals can be switched on by a button held by labouring women and pressed with the onset of contractions.

Sadly, clinical trials assessing whether the TENS machine is indeed effective to counter the pain of labour have thrown up inconclusive results. I've seen it used for many years, and my view is that it can be really helpful at home during the passive phase of labour but is not so flash at countering the full-on pains of active labour. But it is super safe and may be well worth a shot. Women who want one for their upcoming labour will usually need to hire or borrow one in advance. (Unless they intend on purchasing a machine outright. This I do not recommend because it probably won't ever be touched again. After being rolled out for the big day it will probably sit idle in the garage indefinitely, a tangle of electric cords stuffed in the same cardboard box as a crumpled wedding dress housing a content family of hairy arachnids.)

Gate Control Theory may also explain why some women find relief from sterile water injections. During labour, minute amounts of water are injected under the skin around the lower back, forming small blebs. It can be repeated as many times as labouring women request.

Acupuncture is another option. It's not based on Gate Control Theory and doesn't sit within the realms of Western medicine.

The concept is that fine needles are slotted into meridian lines by skilled practitioners. They influence 'qi' or life energy forces. Whether this is really a thing, I don't know. However, if labouring women wish to try acupuncture and it works for them, I am genuinely delighted.

Doulas, candles, music, TENS, water injections. You can see there are many non-drug options and for many women these can work wonders to counter the emotional response to pain and can make the birth experience a happier one. For many these will be enough, especially those blessed with rapid labours.

However, as for sensing the intensity of pain it is probably a fair call to say all these non-drug strategies only take the edge off the pain, at best. For many labouring women, none of these options substantially dull the strong pains that come with active labour.

Drug (or pharmacological) options

In 1847, the anaesthetic power of chloroform was discovered by the Edinburgh physician James Young Simpson, who also happened to be an obstetrician. Around that time, he and his two adventurous assistants (James Matthew Duncan and George Skene Keith) had a somewhat fringe hobby they indulged in during evenings of personally inhaling experimental chemicals. In Simpson's dining room. Their hope was to find one with an anaesthetising effect that was preferably not fatal.

It is unclear whether their self-experimentation was done before dinner or after. If after, they were breathing in mysterious chemicals on a full stomach – something we now know to be very dangerous for anyone who is anaesthetised (if any of them vomited while unconscious they would have inhaled half-digested haggis into their lungs, which would efficiently kill them). And I trust these poisonous experimental chemicals weren't carelessly left unlabelled on the extensive spice rack of the Simpson kitchen.

On 4 November 1847, they tested a chemical called chloroform. It was selected on the flimsy basis that a Robert Glover reported just five years earlier that it could induce sleep in large animals. Never mind that it was widely considered unsafe for humans.

On inhaling the chloroform, they experienced a brief euphoric stage of a 'general mood of cheer and humour' before collectively passing out. It is puzzling why the three intrepid pioneers simultaneously inhaled something that could have wiped them all out. Wouldn't it have been more sensible for Simpson to nominate one of his obliging young assistants to test it out first? Happily, death wasn't to be their fate – the following morning they all regained consciousness.

The moment Simpson awoke he knew he was onto something. Ever the responsible uncle, he did the obvious thing: he rushed up to his young niece Miss Petrie and tried it on her. After inhaling the chloroform his niece dreamily announced, 'I am an angel!' Then passed out. Luckily, for the sake of ongoing sibling harmony among the Simpson family, James' beloved niece managed to wake up. This is just as well since the drug is, in fact, not completely safe as it can induce fatal heart rhythm disturbances. Robert Glover ultimately died of a chloroform overdose, an ironic twist of fate given it was probably he – not Simpson – who actually discovered the anaesthetic potential of the drug but never received the credit (and almost certainly, he became hooked on the euphoric properties of the very stuff he had discovered).

News of the miraculous discovery spread quickly. In that same year of 1847 Queen Victoria, pregnant with her sixth child, caught wind of it and was keen to give it a try. But the wise royal physicians cautioned her against it, so she endured labour without it. When she was pregnant once more in 1850 there was another robust parlay among the royal physicians. Again, they cautioned Queen Victoria that it was not safe to use chloroform. One progressive opinion offered by the obstetrician Professor Charles Meigs was that the painful contractions during labour were 'natural and physiological forces that the Divinity has ordained us (i.e. women, not him) to enjoy or to suffer'. Nice one, Charlie.

However, by her eighth pregnancy in 1853 the tide of opinion had turned. The royal doctors had enough confidence in chloroform's benefits that they agreed to offer it for the forthcoming labour. On Thursday 7 April 1853, Queen Victoria gave birth to Prince Leopold after inhaling chloroform for 53 minutes from a handkerchief. She pronounced it 'delightful beyond measure'.

Some might tsk tsk the conservative attitude of the royal physicians who seemingly deprived the queen of a powerful analgesic agent for two births after its discovery. In contrast I am rather amazed that within six years, an experimental chemical (one with an uncertain safety profile) could progress from its first use in humans to being given to a monarch leading an empire that ruled over a quarter of the world's population (some 450 million subjects). At any rate, chloroform heralded the era of pharmacological therapies to combat the pain of childbirth.

We don't use chloroform today because it is too dangerous (we aren't enthused about giving drugs that can seriously muck about with the rhythmic pumping of mum's heart). Instead, three pharmacological pain relief options are commonly offered in the birth suites of today: inhaled nitrous oxide (popularly known as laughing gas), opiates (such as morphine or pethidine), and epidurals. Of all these pain relief options the epidural is far and away the most effective in removing the sensation of pain during labour.

Nitrous oxide

Nitrous oxide is a safe odourless gas sucked in through a mouthpiece or a mask held by labouring women. The gas used in the birth suite is a 50:50 mix of nitrous oxide and oxygen, and how it dulls pain remains unclear. It is a testament to human ingenuity that we have somehow discovered curiously different uses for the same molecule; not only have we figured out breathing it in can lessen the pain during childbirth and dental work but adding it to fuel adds a massive kick to the engine of high-performance cars (if you need solid proof, just watch *Fast & Furious*). It can even help propel rockets.

For maximum effect there needs to be a good amount of the stuff swirling about in the lungs, where some is absorbed into the bloodstream to reach the brain. Optimally, women start sucking deeply on the mouthpiece around 30 seconds before a contraction, but since the onset of the next contraction can be hard to anticipate most simply start inhaling once they feel the beginnings of the next contraction.

Nitrous oxide makes the person taking it a little disorientated and light-headed as if they are about to faint. Some report a sense of euphoria. Sadly, this most certainly doesn't happen for me – I have given nitrous a try (a rather unspeakable saga of a traumatic shoulder dislocation, self-inflicted while penning this chapter) and was disappointed to feel nothing remotely close to a high.

Once stopped, it wears off in seconds. It may cause nausea but labour itself can do that. Also, no-one can breathe in and push at the same time. This means it cannot be used during the second stage when it is time to push.

It is fair to say nitrous probably takes the edge off strong pain but doesn't take it away altogether. And for some, it has no discernible effect at all. When I sucked it in after my shoulder misadventure the nitrous only made me light-headed and spaced out. But for me it didn't touch the excruciating pain that I now appreciate arises when the bone of one's upper arm is wrenched clean out of the shoulder socket (life hack – don't run down the stairs to take your indoor dog out for a wee. Walk. Doggie can wait).

Still, it may be worth giving nitrous a shot. For those destined for a quick labour it may be an excellent option to tide labouring women over until the cervix is fully dilated and they are ready to push.

Opiates such as morphine

A common option offered during labour is an injection of morphine (or pethidine). These are 'opiate drugs', the same addictive substance that enslaved millions in opium dens during the 19th century. Even today, millions continue to take the stuff recreationally. But don't worry: one or two injections during labour won't get you hooked.

Morphine is isolated from poppy plants whereas pethidine – also known by its technical name meperidine – is synthetically produced. These drugs target the 'opioid' pain receptor on nerve cells sprinkled throughout the brain and spinal cord. They are injected into the muscle of the buttocks or thigh, and their effects last around three to seven hours.

Their advantages are that they can be given quickly and easily. They are usually more effective than nitrous but are still not great at substantially relieving the pains of active labour in full flight. However, they can do a decent job at blunting the severity of labour pain. A scientific paper that gathered all the evidence from many human clinical trials concluded: 'opioids provide some pain relief and moderate satisfaction' (these eight words succinctly sum up an impressively lengthy document chock full of pages upon pages of heavy-going scientific lingo).

However, they can make you sleepy and be relied on to cause nausea and vomiting. To counter this, anti-spew medications are often injected at the same time. These are usually ondansetron (widely known as Zofran) or maxalon; the same friends that have helped many women stagger through their brutally chunderous first trimesters.

Another downside is that they cross the placenta and can make newborns drowsy at birth, so that sometimes a little resuscitation is needed by the paediatric team to initiate breathing. Happily, this sleepiness is short-lived and disappears once the drugs wear off.

For babies born seriously dozy, the paediatric team can give a drug called naloxone to reverse the effects of opiates. Naloxone works well for morphine, but pethidine is broken down into products that hang around for a long time and are not readily reversed by naloxone. Also, pethidine has been linked to lingering effects in the newborn, such as changes in behaviour, more crying (like that's needed) and difficulties taking to the breast. For this reason, many birth suites have moved away from pethidine and now favour morphine, including my own hospital. The United States does not generally use pethidine at all. Perhaps it's time pethidine is retired and morphine is used exclusively.

In short, a morphine (or pethidine) injection may provide some pain relief, is easy to administer (though there is a quick ouchy needle for the recipient) but can cause puking and can make some babies temporarily snoozy at birth. Opiates may be a great choice for some, especially those whose labours are moving along rapidly where a shot of opiates may be all that's needed to tide them along to birth.

Epidural and spinal anaesthesia

The epidural is the only option that decisively removes the pain of labour. It's dramatically effective. Women huffing and puffing before an epidural will often be comfortably seated in bed and soaking in a bit of television after one is put in. Pain free while still in labour – chatting, resting, catching up on sleep. Waiting for full cervical dilation so they can start the business of pushing.

The variation in the rates of epidural uptake across the globe is breathtaking. Seventy per cent of those labouring in the US will have one, but only 36 per cent in the United Kingdom. These are women with presumably similar access to epidurals if they asked for one with the only apparent difference being the land mass they happen to be perched on during labour. Either geographical differences impact on how strongly pain is felt (seriously unlikely) or the astounding difference in uptake is entirely dictated by culture and attitudes.

Many expectant women will have thought a lot about whether they want to have an epidural well before labour happens. And when challenged by the discomfort of active labour, many who initially erred against having one will re-evaluate their choice. What worries me is that I bet many make their choices with a tenuous grasp of the facts, perhaps coloured by a few myths, so I'll spend a fair bit of time exploring the epidural.

The spinal cord dangles down from the base of the brain, like string hanging down from a floating helium balloon (though the spinal cord is not centred but off to one side). It is a thicket of billions of nerves running down from the back of the brain, protected within a hard canal made up of the bony spine. Nerves then splay out of the spinal cord through small gaps studded down the length of the bony spine and these nerves spread out like electrical cabling to reach distant organs and the periphery of the body. The nerves relay information to and fro, between all parts of the body and the brain. Nerves faithfully send commands from brain to muscles so we move, and they bring back signals from the skin to the brain so we can sense.

The spinal cord is wrapped by a protective fibrous layering called the dura (dura mater). Within the encasing of the dura mater the spinal cord is bathed in cerebral spinal fluid, widely known as CSF. Okay, anatomy class is over and I hope you are still with me.

The epidural is an exceptionally thin tube inserted through the lower back into what's called the epidural space. This space is about 5 centimetres deep from the skin surface and just outside the protective coating of the dura. Right next to but not through the dura.

How an epidural is inserted

The midwife or obstetrician will first perform a vaginal examination to make sure the baby isn't really close to being born. Because if it is, there literally may not be time to insert an epidural.

To put in the epidural the labouring woman will be positioned sitting on the bed or lying on her side, back exposed. They will be asked to curl forwards as much as possible, back arched towards the anaesthetist performing the procedure. In this awkward pose, women are then asked to stay still – not the easiest thing to do while being buffeted by waves of painful contractions. But it is important to try as this curled position opens up the tissue spaces in the back, making it easier for the anaesthetist to position the epidural as speedily as possible.

The back is painted with an antiseptic wash. It is usually pink and ice cold. The anaesthetist then numbs a spot on the lower back by injecting a bleb of local anaesthetic just under the skin – a quick sting. An epidural introducer needle is then put into the back through the numbed spot to locate the epidural space by feel. Once found, the tiny epidural tubing is threaded through the inside of the introducer needle and slid into the epidural space. The introducer needle is then whipped out and the epidural tubing left in.

Once in place the epidural catheter – or tubing – which starts in the epidural space in the back, emerges through a tiny hole in the lower back (where the introducer needle once entered), runs up the back towards the shoulder, securely taped on the skin. The tubing continues from the upper back to a machine called a syringe driver. This is attached to a metal pole poking up from one side of the bed (such a pole is an essential prop to denote 'hospital bed' in any respectable Hollywood medical drama). The syringe driver releases very precise amounts of local anaesthetic into the epidural tubing which dribbles out of the other end into the epidural space within the back. This local anaesthetic then seeps into the major nerve endings supplying the uterus, birth canal and legs to provide powerful pain relief. Once in, the epidural is left to run until the baby is born.

Often, the epidural doesn't just block pain but also motor control of the legs. The motor block is usually not absolute, meaning women can still move but they will feel less control. This can make it hazardous to walk about, so those with an epidural may need to lounge in bed for the rest of labour.

A urinary catheter is inserted into the bladder, as women with an epidural will not be able to reliably sense when they need to urinate. Without one, their bladders could fill right up and become damaged by excessive stretch. Finally, for those with an epidural we will continuously monitor fetal heart rate patterns using a cardiotocograph (or CTG).

Within a few hours after the baby is birthed it's removed by simply sliding it out. Muscle control and full sensation promptly returns.

Many women are under the impression that to insert an epidural the anaesthetist needs to perilously dodge the spinal cord dangling just millimetres away from the end of the needle, where a few nervous tremors could result in catastrophic permanent paralysis. This is absolutely not the case. The spinal cord hanging down from the brain ends well above the spot where an epidural is placed. And well clear of the introducer needle.

If a decision is made to perform a caesarean section and an epidural is already in place the anaesthetist can conveniently 'top up' the epidural by squirting in more drugs through the epidural catheter. This 'top-up' takes effect within 10 minutes and provides a far more powerful level of pain (and motor) blockade than the epidural infusion so that a painless operation can be done.

If a caesar is needed but an epidural is not in place then a spinal anaesthetic is often done instead of an epidural. Unlike an epidural where tubing is left in, a spinal anaesthetic is a single shot injection of local anaesthetic agents. The other major difference is that the needle of the spinal anaesthetic pierces the dura mater and delivers the numbing drugs straight into the subarachnoid space where the nerves of the spinal cord are floating about in the cerebral spinal fluid (or CSF).

The pros and cons of an epidural

The massive pro of an epidural is that if it's working well, the pain relief is absolute. As sensory pain removal goes nothing else comes close (except being knocked out). Another compelling pro is that if mum ends up needing a forceps or vacuum birth, having an epidural running will make these procedures far more comfortable. As just mentioned, having one in is convenient if a caesar is ultimately needed as we can simply squirt more drug into the epidural catheter and within minutes we can start the operation.

Of course, something this effective has some risks. There is quite a list. But before we work through them do bear in mind most women having an epidural will not develop any of them. Also, most are a nuisance but are not serious. Serious complications caused by epidurals are exceptionally rare.

I have grouped the potential complications arising from epidural as those that do happen from time to time, those that are uncommon, and lastly those that can be more serious but are also rare.

Firstly, to those that do happen from time to time.

Doesn't work properly: Sometimes the epidural has been slotted in but is not working well (darn it!). It may be providing less pain relief on one side of the body or hardly working at all. This can be just plain annoying. It happens roughly 10 per cent of the time.

To try to fix this the anaesthetist can play around with the amount of drug being given through the infusion pump, enlist gravity by repositioning mum to get more drug seeping over to the side where it's not working well, or gently lengthen or shorten the epidural tube within the back to see whether tweaking helps. If none of this works the only unpalatable choices are to tolerate the pain (often, it's still less pain compared to before the epidural was put in) or to take it out and put another one in.

Drops the blood pressure: The epidural can block the nerves supplying blood vessels, causing them to relax and dilate. This can drop the mother's blood pressure. Unfortunately, sometimes this drop sometimes has the knock-on effect of reducing blood supply to the placenta (and hence the fetus). The fetus suddenly gets less oxygen flow from mum, doesn't like it and this leads to what we call 'fetal distress'. We are alerted to this by observing the sudden appearance of worrying fetal heart rate patterns on the CTG suspiciously timed with a drop in mum's blood pressure that happens soon after an epidural is inserted.

To correct the drop in mum's blood pressure we can pump more fluids into the mum's circulation via a drip in her vein (which is always inserted before we put in the epidural), and if this doesn't solve the issue the anaesthetist can give specialised medications to increase the blood pressure, also through the drip. So, even if a drop in the blood pressure caused by an epidural happens, we can get on top of it. And once the blood pressure is corrected, the fetal condition usually improves and the CTG readout recovers.

Itch, nausea and shivering: An epidural can cause itching. However, most women are pretty happy trading horrid, nasty pain with an itch and are not particularly bothered by it. Nausea and vomiting can also happen. For women taking on a green hue we can inject drugs through the drip to rapidly settle the guts.

Shivering happens and we really don't know why exactly. One theory is that the epidural paralyses nerves that control the diameter of blood vessels in the peripheries of the body (such as the arms and legs). These blood vessels respond by dilating wide open which causes a rush of blood from the mum-to-be's inner core to her surface. This shift in blood can cause her to lose heat, make her feel chilly and start shivering.

The shivering is not dangerous and only lasts awhile. To get women comfortable we simply pile on blankets. I can't promise you the blankets we have on offer will be plush, soft or luxurious, but they will be clean and deliciously warm (I dare say those within the throes of labour won't care whether the blankets are authentic cashmere or not).

Now, on to stuff I rate as 'uncommon', affecting 1–2 per cent of those having an epidural.

Problems passing urine: After the birth some women are unable to fully empty their bladder when the urinary catheter is taken out. To deal with this, we rest the bladder then try again the next day. For the small number who still cannot freely urinate on the second go we may need to send them home with a catheter for up to a week to rest the bladder. After this we try once more, and by then bladder function is almost always back to normal. A nuisance when it occurs but it's not dangerous. Just inconvenient.

A pretty terrible headache: For around 1 per cent of women who have an epidural or spinal anaesthesia, a postdural puncture headache can occur. And I'm afraid it can be a rather wretched one. A fair bit more intense than the throbbing affairs that build up during a stressful day at the office (though they can be pretty ordinary too). A headache is something that women who have just birthed could really do without.

A postdural puncture headache arises from a persistent leak of cerebral spinal fluid through a microscopic hole in the dura mater during the procedure. Such a hole is intentionally made during the routine spinal anaesthetic procedure (so that the medication can be injected into the correct spot) and inadvertently made by the tip of the introducer needle while the epidural tubing is being positioned next to the dura mater.

The headache is worsened by sitting or standing, and is relieved when lying flat. The tiny hole causing all this headachy misery usually seals up on its own, but recovery can take a meandering seven to ten days. In the meantime, painkillers can certainly be taken.

Strangely, taking caffeine apparently helps – it has long fascinated me how anyone figured this out. Taking caffeine may also have a bonus stimulant effect for new mums already struggling with the new reality of little sleep and now burdened with a monster headache. Caffeine certainly does wonders for my (non-postdural puncture) headaches. The caffeine is either taken as a tablet (what's the fun in that?), intravenously (I can see the merits…), or even 'doctor's orders' beverages (the dose required per day is three to four 200 millimetre cups of deliciously brewed coffee, six caffeinated soft drinks … or 14 cans of Coke, which I wouldn't advise).

If the postdural puncture headache is stupidly painful then the anaesthetist can try an epidural blood patch. This can be highly effective. Around 20 millilitres of blood is taken from mum's vein in the arm then injected into the back, around the region of the leaky dura. The hope is that it will form a blood clot that seals the leak in the dura.

Now some really rare stuff that can be serious.

In around 1 in 4000–5000 of spinals and epidurals the anaesthetic drug in the back can somehow mischievously defy gravity and trickle upwards towards the brain. If it soaks the region around the level of the chest it may transiently paralyse nerves coordinating vital functions that we'd all prefer are left alone to do their thing. Such as breathing. Rarely, it can cause a cardiac arrest needing resuscitation. Sounds like scary stuff and I suppose it is. Luckily, we are talking about something super rare; there were only 16 incidences of cardiac arrest caused by spinal or epidurals among 2.3 million pregnancies in the United Kingdom, according to one study. And bear in mind that for those who have majorly lucked out to find themselves one of the 0.000007 per cent who arrests, it absolutely does not mean they will snuff it. Remember this will happen at a hospital brimming with highly trained doctors kitted out with medical gear. Mum can be supported until the effects wear off (needless to say, turning off the epidural would be high on the list of management steps). However, things could get a little dramatic if cardiorespiratory resuscitation is needed, as well as other emergency measures. A frightening event unlikely to feature in anyone's birth plan.

Another rare thing that can happen is that an abscess – a small, infected pocket of nasty bacteria and pus – can growth in the epidural space where the epidural tubing once resided. Or in the dura where the spinal needle passed through. It is a pretty delicate spot for an infection and can occasionally cause serious problems, but it can be usually treated effectively with antibiotics which results in a complete recovery.

Now, let's look at some things widely thought to be caused by the epidural (the internet is rife with this stuff) that, in fact, objective research studies examining many thousands of cases haven't managed to confirm a link.

Firstly, the spot where the epidural was placed may throb for a few days, but there is no evidence that epidurals cause a permanent backache. Secondly, many worry about the risk of permanent paralysis. It's an understandable fear as women put two and two together in their mind: needle going into back… hang on a sec, isn't the spinal cord also lurking there somewhere? Reassuringly, there is either no link between an epidural and permanent paralysis, or it's incredibly rare. This makes sense since the epidural catheter is inserted well clear of the spinal cord itself. And the effects of all the anaesthetic drugs we inject are transient. According to one reputable medical source it is so rare that they were unable to hazard a guess as to how often it even happens after an epidural. Now that has got to be reassuring. Many anaesthetists will tell women as part of informed consent for an epidural that there is a tiny risk of permanent paralysis from the back down, then quote a really low figure, typically one in 100,000–200,000.

There is a slightly higher risk of a type of nerve injury called a 'foot drop', but it's still rare (1 in 20,000 to 1 in 40,000 risk). This is where there is difficulty lifting the front part of the foot. It can be permanent. Importantly, those affected can still walk about, but the front of the foot may drag down a bit.

Overall, it is pretty safe to say from large epidemiological studies that the risk of permanent paralysis after an epidural or spinal anaesthetic is tiny.

There is most definitely a rumour actively promulgated – one that has been bouncing about for eons – that a major downside of an epidural is that it increases the chances of medical interventions such as forceps or caesarean sections. This is so widely regarded to be universal truth that many birth classes of today (and of tomorrow) have educators declaring, 'Have an epidural at your peril as it will slow labour and ratchet up your chances of a forceps or a caesarean section. Sure, have one if you really can't bear the pain but it will rob you of a dream natural birth.' In fact, an objective look at the medical evidence has not uncovered a convincing link between an epidural and an increased risk of medical interventions.

One of the highest levels of synthesising medical evidence is a rigid scientific method called a systematic meta-analysis.

It gathers all the published scientific evidence on a topic via a meticulous, systematic search strategy. Using a strict (and dispassionate) statistical approach, the results of all these studies are combined to answer important clinical questions. They can be pretty boring to do (luckily, there are altruistic folk out there who are willing to do them for our benefit, such as enthusiastic junior members of my research team), but the method makes a lot of sense. For example, the larger studies with more participants will more heavily sway the findings.

A systematic meta-analysis published in 2018 combined the findings of many studies and tallied the outcomes of over 10,000 pregnancies. The results were clear: having an epidural was not associated with higher rates of caesars compared with epidural free labours (in this study the comparator group were those opting for opioids instead of an epidural). Reassuringly, the study also concluded having an epidural did not up the risk of having an instrumental birth either (forceps or vacuum birth).

Many will be rather surprised by this. And I suspect many health professionals who work in birth suites simply won't believe these results and will continue informing women that epidurals increase their risk of medical interventions. I understand why this may be; we have all seen women with long labours offered an epidural only to wind up with a caesarean section many hours after. However, even decades of personal clinical experience accumulated by one doctor or midwife cannot match the objective analysis of evidence from 10,000+ women to credibly dispute the objective findings of this important 2018 research study.

To summarise, the big advantage of an epidural is that it can powerfully quash the pains of childbirth. Also, having a working epidural can make instrumental births more comfortable if they are needed. And if a caesar is required, a drug 'top-up' can be conveniently added into the epidural before the procedure.

The drawbacks are that women cannot freely move about the birth suite, and will need a drip in the vein and a catheter in their bladder. They may shiver, itch or spew. Other risks that are uncommon include a drop in the blood pressure, a wretched headache lasting days or difficulties urinating in the days following childbirth. There is a tiny risk of foot drop and a vanishingly small risk of permanent paralysis.

All in all, epidurals and spinal anaesthetics really are very safe. Recent studies have failed to confirm a common belief that it leads to more caesars, forceps or vacuum births (though some will never be convinced of this).

It really does suck that humans are constructed in a way where labour really hurts. It would have been so much more convivial if instead, uterine contractions felt like a tight squeeze and relaxation without all the needless pain thrown in (I can't see why that wouldn't work). But sadly, that's not the case.

However, there are diverse options to deal with the pain of labour which we have now covered: from pretend flickering candles to opium extracts from poppy plantations; AC/DC to aromatherapy; TENS machines to inhaling a similar gas that rev-heads use to add kick to their hotted-up automobiles. Of course, there is also the epidural.

Before we move to the main event – labour – can I impart two final thoughts? Firstly, it is absolutely okay for women to play it by ear and not make firm decisions beforehand. For those who feel this option is for them, I trust this chapter will be particularly useful as it provides sound knowledge to make informed pain relief choices on the fly.

Secondly, the choice of pain relief rests solely with the labouring woman. If this is you, please remember this. If you decide an epidural is what you want, go for it (I support you). Cast aside strident views voiced by friends and family during the pregnancy. And if you are a support person, offer your thoughts if asked, but leave the decision to the person actually trying to give birth. And enthusiastically endorse her choice.

Recap: **Options for pain relief**

1. Pain is both an unpleasant emotional and sensory experience. Countering the emotional response is important and explains why many drug-free strategies are effective. As for the sensory experience of pain, most options take the edge off the pain (to varying degrees). An epidural is the only option that entirely removes the sensation of pain.
2. There are a host of drug-free options that women can try. For many, these are all that's needed, especially those blessed with a rapid labour. They include having trusted support people in the room (birth partner, friends, family, a doula), altering the ambience of the room (candles, music, aromatherapy), breathing techniques, bouncing on a birth ball, adopting different positions, a bath or shower, water injections into the lower back, acupuncture or a TENS machine.
3. The skilled midwife can work with labouring women to try out some of these options.
4. Inhaling nitrous oxide (or 'laughing gas') is an option that works well for some. It's very safe but its effectiveness is variable. Sucked in during contractions, it can elicit light-headedness or even euphoria (for some lucky ones).
5. An injection of an opiate-based drug (mainly morphine) is a pharmacological option. There is good evidence that opiates can blunt the sensory experience of pain, but they commonly

cause vomiting (we administer anti-spew drugs to counter this). Also, they can cross the placenta, making some newborns a little drowsy at birth. At times it will mean the baby needs a little resuscitation at birth, but it's often short-lived and the baby perks right up when the drug wears off.

6. The epidural is the only option that decisively removes the pain of labour. A seriously thin tube is inserted low down in the back (well clear of the nerve bundle that is the spinal cord) and medication is continuously dribbled in. It is left to run until labour is over.

7. Women having an epidural will need an intravenous drip, and a catheter to keep their bladder empty. Also, most will be lounging in bed as the epidural can affect control of the legs.

8. Epidurals are very safe but there are some risks. The more common ones are that it doesn't work properly; causes a transient drop in mum's blood pressure (which can sometimes upset the baby, but we can correct it); and it can cause itching, shivering or vomiting. Less common side effects include a terrible headache and difficulty passing urine in the days following birth. Permanent footdrop is rare (1 in 40,000) and permanent paralysis is stupidly rare.

9. It is reassuring that studies haven't found a link between epidurals and an increased risk of medical procedures such as forceps, ventouses or caesars.

Chapter 3

Warming up the engine: going into labour spontaneously or with a little help

Thanks for sticking around. By this time, I hope readers feel like they are prising open the mysterious black box that is the birth suite – that mystical place where pregnant women step in, the doors close, stuff happens, and they emerge cradling a small human. One that squawks a lot, is not one bit continent and is infuriatingly partial to late night snacking. But precious and loved the moment it arrives.

Chapter 1 provided a bird's eye view of birth: the major players (placenta, uterus, baby), a timeline of events and an overview of what happens in the birth suite. In Chapter 2, we mulled over the various choices on offer to counter the pain of labour. Over the next few chapters, we will finally turn to the task at hand. Labour.

This chapter covers how labour begins. I talk about the fascinating shape-shifting process of 'cervical ripening', a prelude to active labour. I look at strategies widely believed to kickstart natural labour, from eating spicy foods to vigorous exercise, acupuncture and even guzzling castor oil. And pause to reflect how effective they really are. I also walk through how we induce labour, where we kickstart proceedings instead of waiting for labour to start spontaneously. Induced labour is now really common and therefore well worth knowing about. The chapter that follows is really a continuation of this one and tackles full blown labour.

Exciting. We are hurtling towards the business end of childbirth.

Cervical ripening: preparing for the big day

I attended Kilsyth East Primary School for seven years of my life, a forgettable public school hidden in the eastern outskirts of Melbourne. Even more forgettable and hidden now as it no longer exists. No-one has even felt moved to pen a Wikipedia entry in homage. In fact, its web footprint is barely existent – the top hit on a Google search is titled: 'Lost schools of the 1990s'. In 1984 we memorably buried a time capsule with a lavish ceremony. Originally slated for re-opening in 2034 to stoke joyous wonderment among an unborn future generation (50 years after its concrete incarceration) I am guessing our loser time capsule suffered an undignified premature exit from its concrete tomb to make way for affordable suburban housing. I have no idea where it is languishing right now. Perhaps shoved in a dark filing cabinet at the local public library, just a precariously short step from being tossed into landfill with the next council approved library renovation. Losing it will be an affront to humanity because priceless artistic treasures contained within will perish along with it, such as artwork from Mr Thiele's grade four class (one of which is mine).

For those seven years of schooling I was driven to Kilsyth East Primary School by Auntie Alice, a parent of my friend at the time and our neighbour. Every morning we would sit in her circa 1970s Toyota Celica with its distinctive matte gold finish. She would turn on the engine and leave it running for 10 or so minutes to warm up. Then we drove off (Auntie Alice is not her real name, of course. And she wasn't my real aunt either. It's an Asian thing to respectfully call anyone of the next generation 'auntie').

During the minutes sitting in the car waiting for the Celica's engine to warm up, we'd merrily chat. They were such lovely chats. I still recall sitting in the car in the small indoor garage, the sweet fumes from the exhaust enveloping us and seeping into our young pre-teen lungs. It was also an era when petrol contained lead. I probably still harbour millions of microscopic souvenirs from that cherished era of childhood scattered throughout my neural circuits. I hold them personally responsible for my permanent inability to recall names. But do not get me wrong – Auntie Alice was an amazingly generous person who took in a new Asian migrant boy under her care. For seven years she got me to where I needed, to be educated. It is difficult to find such saints these days.

Auntie Alice's circa 1970s Toyota Celica needed a preparation step to function optimally. First, the engine needed to warm up. Engine on, gears on neutral, car not moving. Unlike the magical vehicles of today, cars belonging to previous generations needed a warm engine to run efficiently. Once warm, the car was ready for driving. This is a (very) rough analogy that could be applied to the uterus as it prepares for birth. From a standing start the uterus cannot snap into full flight active labour within moments. Instead, the uterus also goes through a preparation step so that it's primed for the dramas of active labour. But it doesn't do this by warming up some motor. Instead, its preparation step is an amazing process where the cervix undergoes a remarkable transformation called 'cervical ripening'.

The cervix approaches the final weeks of pregnancy in the same configuration that it had been throughout pregnancy – in the 'unripe' state. An unripe cervix is clamped shut with no possibility of letting a baby pass. Being unripe therefore serves an incredibly important role keeping the developing ball of cute and cuddly securely held within the uterus for many months (until it is ready to emerge and take on critical baby responsibilities – such as regurgitating half-digested milk onto daddy's freshly pressed shirt. And onto his designer tie. And down his neck). If the cervix ripens too early it can lead to premature birth, something that we'd really prefer to avoid.

The shape of an unripe cervix is a cylinder between 2.5 and 5 centimetres long. We know this as we can readily measure its length by ultrasound. It has a firm consistency to the touch and there is a tiny tunnel running through its centre, called the cervical canal. This canal joins the inner cavity of the uterus to the birth canal, or the vagina. While the cervix is unripe, the cervical canal is so narrow it could barely accommodate a chubby worm to wriggle through (no matter how motivated it may be), let alone a baby.

Any time from around 37 weeks gestation the cervix starts to ripen. It transforms from being cylindrical to a thin opening that is 2–3 centimetres wide, and soft and stretchy (we assess cervical ripeness by performing a vaginal examination with a gloved hand).

A few things happen as the cervix ripens. The cylinder shortens in length and when it reaches the thinness of cloth, we deem the cervix 'fully effaced'. It also changes in consistency from 'firm' (feels like cooked calamari) to 'soft' (with an uncanny feel of uncooked calamari). The cervical canal opens from being 'closed' (where the hole is so tiny it cannot accommodate a finger on the examiners gloved hand) to 2 or 3 centimetres dilated (where the examiner can easily pass a gloved finger through the cervix to tap the head of the unborn baby). Cervical ripening can happen in the absence of labour or can evolve over hours during the passive stage of early labour.

Thus, an unripe cervix is a little like a cylindrical segment of rubber piping with a tiny hole running through it. A ripe cervix is a little like elastic-rimmed leg holes found in some long pyjamas or tracksuit pants – thin and stretchy (but smaller scale, of course). Once the cervix has ripened, it is primed and ready for labour.

There are three reasons why cervical ripening is useful to know about:

It explains why the mythical 'mucous' plug can appear as women approach their due date. As the cervix dilates during ripening a mucous plug topples out from the cervical canal, where it had been contently wedged in for months. This is widely known as losing the mucous plug. It plops out onto the underwear as a sticky, stringy, goopy blob that may be variably bloodstained. With a remarkably similar consistency to snot. This vivid analogy is not my crass invention but widely used in the clinic where pregnant women are asked whether the blob was stringy, like snot. A 'yes' is taken as evidence it was probably the mucous plug.

It can be thrilling for women to see the mucous plug emerge because many are under the impression that active labour will inevitably follow. Losing the plug does indeed increase the chances that labour will fire up soon as it often means the cervix is ripening. But I am sorry to say it is no sure bet. There have been many who have seen their mucous plug tumble out but dismayed to find themselves stubbornly pregnant weeks afterwards. Conversely, most women go into labour without ever laying eyes on their mucous plug.

The second point of interest is that for those who are not in labour but are nearing their due date, the riper the cervix the more likely that labour will happen soon (irrespective of any sighting of the mucous plug). For this reason, women close to their expected date of birth women can request a vaginal examination to assess how ripe their cervix is, to get a rough guestimate whether labour may be close. Although a ripe cervix does increase the likelihood of going into labour sooner (compared to having an unripe cervix) it is also no guarantee. Those with an unripe cervix can still go into active labour within days.

The last thing to say about cervical ripeness is that the riper the cervix at the start of labour the more likely it will smoothly progress to a vaginal birth. This is why when we induce labour, we take steps to ripen the cervix before we switch on actual labour, something we will discuss very soon.

The simple take-home messages on cervical ripeness: the riper the better, and goop is good (aka the mucous plug).

Well-known strategies to kickstart spontaneous labour...that probably don't work

Women beyond 37 weeks pregnant are waiting. On waking each morning, they ponder whether this will be the day. Understandably, many will interrogate Google to hunt for cunning tricks to kickstart labour. And they are likely to collide into the same tired list that has bounced around for decades: castor oil, vigorous walking, raspberry leaf tea, more sex and spicy food. And acupuncture. They are all safe (and some delicious); however, the evidence is slim at best that any of these reliably bring on labour.

In the case of castor oil, the tenuous theory holds that for those who manage to scull the stuff (and keep it swallowed), the oil will incite hideous bowel symptoms – loose bowel motions, diarrhoea and vomiting. Somehow, whipping the bowels into a gaseous, gurgling frenzy is thought to persuade its quiet neighbour – the uterus – that it really ought to awake from its slumber and start contracting. Sadly, although drinking straight castor oil will no doubt get the bowels really annoyed, I do not think it gets the uterus going. I suspect the uterus doesn't really give a fig how gurgly and unsettled the bowels are. One account on the history of castor oil observed that it was freely prescribed from 1931 until 1948 to induce labour but fell out of favour 'due to the side effects of violent diarrhoea, resulting in patient exhaustion'. Sounds messy. For those who still wish to give it a crack, go for it by all means but do keep a toilet handy. And perhaps keep the hair in a high ponytail.

The theory behind gobbling spicy foods to kickstart labour is probably similar to castor oil (set off the bowels…set off the womb). For those visiting an Indian restaurant while heavily pregnant, I hope you enjoy the meal. You deserve it. But I personally think it is unnecessary to set your tongue (and innards) ablaze by ordering the hottest available tikka masala.

And I am not sure how more sex and vigorous walking is meant to set off labour. Presumably crude shaking physically jolts the uterus into action. But given both can be safely done during the long months of pregnancy without activating preterm labour (which is a good thing), it seems unlikely to me that these activities would suddenly acquire the superpower to trigger labour simply because women have reached term gestation. Interestingly, whether sex can precipitate natural labour was put to the test in a clinical trial by an adventurous Malaysian research team. They persuaded highly obliging couples to be randomly allocated by the researchers to have regular sex or to abstain (which I am sure heavily pregnant women did not mind one bit). Sadly, the study did not find sex kicked off labour.

I have a theory as to why something as bizarre as raspberry leaf tea has wheedled its way onto the common list of strategies to start natural labour. If you think about it, it's a pretty niche tea (it's not even the potentially delicious raspberry but the leaf). And it's generally not a feature of anyone's weekly grocery list. My pet conspiracy theory is that raspberry leaf tea is the by-product of a cunning marketing strategy of yesteryear – its labour-inducing properties entirely made up to sell seriously underperforming tea. Whether or not I have uncovered a major scam, I do not think that raspberry leaf tea – as delectable as the brew may be – really helps women go into labour.

As for acupuncture, it depends on the existence of meridian lines and qi energy that can neither be seen, felt or detected in any way nor explained by conventional science. So, although safe, acupuncture lies beyond the realm of conventional medicine.

I would like to head off a chorus of outrage that may be stirring in the hearts of many who have had positive experiences from these strategies. The fact is that once pregnancies have reached

38 weeks gestation, the chances that labour will spontaneously kick in at any moment sharply rise over the ensuing weeks. Therefore, if the uterus starts contracting the very night of a flavoursome lamb vindaloo with extra chilli, no-one can tell for certain whether it was all due to Mrs Patel's superb cooking or it was just coincidence. This is anecdotal evidence. But, of course, for experienced mums who are adamant that a brisk walk around the hilly seaside, a scrumptious curry or a late afternoon rumble in a sun-dappled boudoir got them into labour I am not going to take this cherished memory from them. All these strategies are very safe for those who wish to try them. With the possible exception of ingesting spicy foods or castor oil as these may generate noisy tummy rumbling and unpleasant volatile gases – side effects that may adversely impact on the auditory and olfactory wellbeing of those around them.

Stretch and sweep

A 'stretch and sweep' is one very simple technique to get women into spontaneous labour that may actually work. While performing a vaginal examination, the examiner places a gloved finger into the cervical canal and performs a few circumferential sweeps. The examiner's finger will be in contact with the fetal head sitting adjacent at the other end of the cervical opening, though placental membranes overlying the head prevents direct contact.

A stretch and sweep can only be done if the cervix is sufficiently dilated to accommodate the examiner's finger – at least a centimetre open. The theory behind the stretch and sweep is that it may stir some sort of biological or hormonal response that accelerates cervical ripening, or even trigger labour. It can be uncomfortable for some, but many women tolerate a stretch and sweep just fine. Also, it is pretty quick. Those finding it too disagreeable can simply ask the examiner to stop.

Women should not be alarmed if there is a small amount of fresh vaginal bleeding soon after the stretch and sweep (or, in fact, after any internal examination) as it is almost certainly a small harmless trickle from the wall of the cervical canal and not from within the uterus.

There is evidence that stretch and sweeps are effective in stirring up labour. A meta-analysis (a scientific study that combines data from many clinical studies) that reported the outcomes of just under 3000 pregnancies concluded a stretch and sweep reduces the chance of reaching 41 weeks gestation still pregnant. As a sort of bonus, the same study also found that for women who did go into spontaneous labour, those who had had a stretch and sweep beforehand may score shorter labours. This is plausible if the stretch and sweep helps trigger the cervix to ripen.

A stretch and sweep is an option for those nearing their due date, but it only works sometimes and cannot be relied on to trigger labour. However, it is safe and well worth a shot.

Why we induce labour

Induction of labour is a process where the clinical team gets labour started instead of everyone waiting for spontaneous (or 'natural') labour to happen. It is most commonly offered for medical reasons. And, on occasion, women simply request it.

There are two steps to inducing labour. Firstly, if unripe the cervix needs ripening. This is done by either inserting a balloon just inside the opening of the cervix (mechanical ripening) or placing a hormone called prostaglandin in the vagina close to the cervix (hormonal ripening). Once the cervix is ripe, we then start active contractions by administering another hormone called oxytocin into the mum's circulation through a drip in her vein. The microscopic oxytocin particles latch onto the surface of the uterus and issues forth the command to contract.

Induced labour is really common. For example, in 2017 around 43 per cent of pregnancies in Australia reaching at least 37 weeks of pregnancy had labour induced. Around the same time, 32 per cent pregnancies had labour induced in the United Kingdom. This means many reading this book will end up having their labour induced or will be supporting someone who will. Therefore, we'll spend a bit of time on this important topic.

There are many medical reasons why women are offered an induction of labour. One important example of a fetal reason to induce labour is when the clinical team harbours suspicions that baby is small and undergrown in the womb, a condition called fetal growth restriction. It's picked up by ultrasound. The concern is that fetal growth restriction can reflect a placenta that is dangerously under-functioning. This means if we patiently wait for spontaneously labour to happen, there is a risk for a small number of these affected pregnancies that the placenta will stop working entirely, leading to a stillbirth. Therefore, once a pregnancy with fetal growth restriction arrives at a sufficiently mature gestation (we aim for about 38 weeks gestation, depending on how small the baby is) it is probably safer for the dainty munchkin to be birthed sooner rather than later. Once out of the womb, the growth-restricted baby no longer relies on its under-functioning (and possibly failing) placenta to breathe. Instead, it switches over to its own lungs and the stillbirth risk evaporates.

One important example of a maternal reason to induce labour is when the pregnancy is affected by a condition called preeclampsia. This arises when a diseased placenta has the indecency to spill noxious proteins into mum's bloodstream. They circulate widely, injuring mum's blood vessels throughout her body and causing high blood pressure. Many organs supplied by these damaged blood vessels can then become majorly sick: important ones too, such as mum's liver, kidney, lungs and even her brain. Occasionally, the maternal organ injury wrought by preeclampsia can be life-endangering. Delivery effectively cures mum of her preeclampsia because it rids her of the diseased placenta rudely pouring disagreeable proteins into her circulation. Finally free of the continuing insult, mum's blood vessels and her organs can heal in peace.

These are just two examples – there are many other reasons why we may recommend an induction of labour.

The ARRIVE trial: is inducing labour safe?

For decades it had been universally accepted as hard fact that being induced carries a major drawback: that it doubles the risk of a caesarean section compared to patiently waiting for spontaneous labour to kick in. Many still believe this.

The world of obstetrics and midwifery was rocked by the findings of a landmark scientific report published in 2018 – an epic clinical trial almost without precedence in its scale. Its findings upended conventional wisdom.

The study, called the 'ARRIVE trial', recruited just over 6000 altruistic mothers-to-be in their first pregnancy. They were randomly allocated to be either induced when they reached 39 weeks gestation or to keep waiting for spontaneous labour to set in and only be induced if they reached 41 weeks gestation still pregnant.

The ARRIVE trial decisively showed inducing labour at 39 weeks is safe. The surprising thing was that being deliberately induced at this earlier gestation actually decreased the chances of having a caesar, compared to waiting for natural labour to set in: a shocking finding that provoked gasps from obstetricians and midwives around the world. (This actually happened. I was in a packed auditorium among thousands of eager ears in Dallas when the results were first revealed at a major scientific conference. I distinctly heard a ripple of gasps when the main findings were announced – with a touch of American flare. I didn't gasp, only because I am not a gasper. If I were, I am sure I would have gasped too).

The shocks did not end there. The trial also hinted that for those arriving at 39 weeks gestation undelivered, inducing labour instead of waiting for it to happen may actually be safer for the baby. The findings regarding the baby's health were not conclusive – you'd need to conduct an even huger trial to prove it – but the point is, induction did not increase the risk of serious health issues challenging the newborn during the few weeks after its birth.

Finally, women randomly allocated to be induced at 39 weeks gestation actually reported lower pain scores than those who waited for spontaneous labour. This dispels another long-cherished belief that continues to make the rounds on the web – that induced labours are more painful than those that come on naturally. Surprisingly, those who were induced also reported they felt more in control during childbirth compared to those who waited.

Let me try to clarify a point here. The findings of the trial do not say being induced is always better than going into labour naturally. The best thing is to go into spontaneous labour just before the due date as this has the lowest chance of needing medical interventions. But going into natural labour isn't a choice: it either happens or doesn't. What the ARRIVE trial is saying is that for those who have reached 39 weeks and haven't gone into labour (and therefore still pregnant), booking an induction rather than venturing past the due date does not appear to be harmful. And possibly a tad beneficial.

The findings of the ARRIVE trial have left our heads spinning. For decades we accepted as fact that we better have a good reason to induce someone because we upped their risk of a caesar. Now we are not so sure. In fact, the ARRIVE trial suggests being induced at 39 weeks gestation actually drops the chances of winding up with a caesar (but only by a little bit), compared to waiting beyond this gestation for labour to set in. The pain is no worse. And it seems safe for the baby, possibly safer.

I suggest society is nowhere near the point of inducing everyone at 39 weeks gestation. And perhaps should never be. However, I think it's a safe bet that the mighty ARRIVE trial will cause rates of inductions to soar over coming years. This is because the results are going to lower the threshold for inductions to be offered as there are no apparent downsides. And for women requesting to be induced at 39 weeks of pregnancy as their preferred birth plan there is no longer a sound medical basis to refuse it.

The first step to inducing labour – ripen the cervix

Cervical ripeness is assessed via a gentle internal examination by the doctor or midwife at an antenatal visit close to the day of the planned induction. Those lucky enough to be endowed with a ripe cervix – soft, a few centimetres dilated and thinned out – can bypass the ripening step. They only need to come on the actual day of the planned induction to have their baby. For those with an unripe cervix, we need to ripen it before we can get active labour going. As mentioned, having the cervix as ripe as possible at the start of labour maximises the chances of a smooth passage to a vaginal birth.

Cervical ripening is done a day or two before we start active labour and there are two ways to do it: hormonal or mechanical. Both are commonly done.

Hormonal ripening

For hormonal ripening we insert hormone preparations deep into the vagina near the cervix, the target organ. Hormones are microscopic molecules that bind onto 'receptors' studded on the surface of cells and tissues throughout the body including, of course, the cervix. We all have hundreds of different receptors that each recognise just one or a few hormones and ignores all others. Receptors are primed to switch on whenever a hormone it recognises latches onto it. Once in the 'on' state the receptor fires up an elegant molecular signalling relay system to perform specific tasks, such as instructing the cervix to ripen. Hence, hormones and their receptors throughout the body work as a 'lock and key' signalling system.

It's a little like when a wife makes the grim discovery that dishes their other half had promised to dry an hour ago are still perched on the dishes rack suspiciously sodden. The wife (the hormone in the analogy) who made the unwelcome find floats about the house with purpose until she locates her husband (the receptor) and sends an exquisitely clear signal (the beauty of this graceful biological system is that the signal doesn't even need words. Just folded arms and a piercing gaze is sufficient). The receptor is activated and springs into action; they pause their favourite Netflix series, head off to the kitchen and hunt for a tea towel (while assiduously avoiding eye contact). And the job gets done.

Note the elegant specificity of this system. Both 'hormone' and 'receptor' will only react to very specific hormones or receptors (such as spouse or partner, mother and mother-in-law), while ignoring most others (like cat, puppy, naggy neighbour, to-do list or someone else's bratty child).

Hormones that send the order to the cervix to ripen are called 'prostaglandins'. The prostaglandins we use to ripen the cervix are identical to those involved in natural cervical ripening. We are simply adding the prostaglandins artificially to hasten the process.

There are a few prostaglandin preparations. Prostin is a gel preparation that's squirted into the vagina via a blunt plastic syringe. When positioned, a plunger is pushed and a gel mixed with prostaglandin leaks out the other end into the vagina, gooping up the region near the cervix. Prostin is usually applied once or twice (spaced six to eight hours apart).

Another hormone option called misoprostol is a small tablet that's inserted into the vagina or even taken orally. Cervadil is yet another type – a thin strip of material infused with prostaglandin.

It is slid inside the vagina via an internal examination and gently placed as close to the cervix as possible. The other end of the material runs along the length of the vagina and dangles just outside the vaginal opening. It is left in for 12 hours and removed by pulling on the strip extending out the vaginal opening.

Mechanical ripening

The second broad approach to ripen the cervix is mechanical ripening. Sounds intimidatingly machine-like but it's nothing of the sort. We place a balloon filled with 30–50 millilitres of fluid inside the lower end of the uterus, just above the cervix, where it's left for 12–24 hours.

The device many of us use is a Foley's catheter, the same catheter we put into bladders during surgery to keep it empty of urine. A Foley's catheter is made of flexible latex tubing around 30 centimetres long and only 5 millimetres wide. It is therefore thin enough to comfortably thread through the cervical canal even if it is in the unripe state and the opening is very narrow. An inflatable balloon sits at the tip of the latex tubing.

To insert the balloon, we often position women in leg supports known as stirrups. The stirrups are padded supports that sit just under the calves of the leg. With women lying on their backs, the stirrups rotate open the thighs so the clinician putting in the balloon can access the vaginal opening. We gently pass a speculum into the vagina, the same one used to perform pap smears. The speculum holds the walls of the vagina off to the sides so we can see the cervix.

We thread the tip of the Foley's catheter through the cervical canal. Once through the cervix, the balloon at the tip of the catheter tubing is inflated with water (added by squirting it into the other end of the long flexible tubing). When inflated the balloon is about the size of half a fist. Placental membranes prevent direct contact between the balloon and the baby's head.

Once the balloon is in position the flexible tubing on the other end of the catheter is taped onto mum's inner thigh. Mum is then free to move about and the tubing does not hinder number ones or twos. Many hospitals will send women home with the balloon in, to return the next day for the actual induction. Happily, having the balloon inside is surprisingly pain free. Some feel some minor pelvic cramping which disappears, but most feel nothing at all.

After 12–24 hours the balloon is deflated and the catheter easily slides out. Hopefully, the balloon has weaved its magic and has ripened the cervix so we can start active labour.

An alternative to the Foley's catheter is a Cook's catheter. It has two balloons: one that sits inside the cervix – just like the Foley's catheter – and a second balloon in the vagina. So, when in place the cervix is wedged between the two balloons. It's fancier than the Foley's catheter – two balloons, not one – but it's unclear whether the Cook's catheter is more effective (though I am sure the manufacturer swears by it). One advantage it does have over the Foley's catheter is that it's latex free for those who are allergic.

It is uncertain how balloon ripening works, but there is likely to be more to it than simply jamming open the cervix by force. The stretch that the balloon exerts on the cervix probably stimulates local production and release of prostaglandins, which then activates receptors to ripen the cervix. Whatever it does, it works.

Pros and cons of the hormonal and mechanical methods

An advantage of hormonal methods to ripen the cervix is that they are easier to insert than balloons. But let me stress that most women tolerate the balloon insertion just fine. A few may find the insertion uncomfortable, and a small number cannot tolerate it at all. If we are unable to put in a balloon, we can always revert to hormone options.

A major advantage of the balloon catheter is that it hardly ever causes uterine contractions. Most feel barely anything while it's in, and they have a better chance of getting a restful sleep before the big day. In contrast, hormonal methods can often cause the uterus to irregularly contract but not go into labour. This causes repetitive crampy pain which can be quite trying, especially overnight when the poor woman is trying to get some decent shut-eye before the big day. Mum-to-be may need pain relief medications to get through the night. And perhaps even a sleeping tablet.

On occasion the hormone-ripening methods cause overly long contractions or contractions that occur too often. This is called 'hyperstimulation', and this is not particularly normal nor desirable. Some unborn babies do not take kindly to this: they fail to get the oxygen they need with these abnormal uterine contractions and become unwell. We are alerted to this by the appearance of very abnormal fetal heart rate patterns on the cardiotocograph. On occasion, the fetal heart rate patterns are so concerning that we are forced to do an emergency caesarean section because of fetal distress. In contrast, the balloon catheter usually doesn't provoke uterine contractions meaning it is less likely to cause this problem. For this reason, over the past decade many birth suites have shifted from hormonal methods to balloon catheters as the preferred choice to ripen the cervix (including my own hospital).

Don't worry if the birth suite caring for the pregnancy you are involved in prefers to use hormonal methods of cervix ripening over the balloon. Both are very safe.

Unfortunately, neither method always works. Some uncooperative cervices remain stubbornly unripe after many attempts. Although this doesn't happen very often it is enormously frustrating when it does. One option is to progress to the next step of starting up active contractions anyway using the oxytocin drip, although the chances of a successful vaginal birth when starting off with a very unripe cervix is far lower than if the cervix is ripe. The second option is to persist trying to ripen the cervix such as inserting another balloon or giving more and more hormonal preparations, until we have maxed out on the amount we can safely give. But if the cervix hasn't willingly ripened on the first go, it often won't readily do so with subsequent tries.

The second step to inducing labour – breaking the waters and starting active labour

Finally. After a seemingly never-ending pregnancy that bubbled along with aching hips, tingly hands, a shift of one's centre of gravity, a blocked left ear, thrush, clogged bowels, swollen feet and a decent quantity of saliva-laced chunder, the long-awaited day of the planned induction is upon us. The cervix is ripe and we are set.

To get active labour going we 'break the waters' then run the hormone oxytocin through a drip in a vein which gets the uterus contracting.

The waters are broken by using an instrument called an amnihook (or something similar) to pierce a hole in the placental membranes. These carpet the inner walls of the uterus and cross over the cervix. They form a humungous watertight bag that holds the baby dreamily floating around in a deliciously warm amniotic fluid bath throughout pregnancy (we call the membranes 'plural' because there are two layers, called the amnion and the chorion. Being right next to each other they can almost be considered as one).

Let me reassure you that the amnihook is not scary. It's made of plastic, has a friendly yellow colour, is around 30 centimetres long, and the 'hook' on the end that is used to scratch a hole in the placental membranes is just a small nub of plastic that isn't really very sharp. If scrapped on the skin of your arm it might eke out a few pathetic white scratches as sharp fingernails might but would struggle to draw blood. Thus, breaking the waters does not hurt you or the baby. Also, the membranes are very thin and are easily pierced.

Holding the amnihook with the left hand, the midwife or doctor performs an internal examination with their right hand to tent open the cervix and guide the instrument through to abut the placental membranes. We then do a few scrapes of the amnihook on the membranes until amniotic fluid flows out of the vagina, which is the tell-tale sign the membranes are ruptured. Often, it's a small trickle but other times an impressive gush (that soaks the recently laundered pants of the hapless obstetrician performing the procedure).

We then insert a drip (intravenous cannula) into the vein so we can run a slow infusion of a drug called oxytocin to switch on active contractions. A drip is 1–2 centimetres of fine plastic tubing slotted into a vein, and we usually choose one on the back of the hand, on the wrist or a juicy vein in the bend of the forearm. A needle is needed to pierce through the skin in order to reach the vein, then it's removed and only fine tubing is left.

We administer drugs and fluids through drips because they can rapidly reach the bloodstream and act quickly. Also, we can be very precise in controlling the dose of drug that reaches the circulation.

Oxytocin is a hormone released from the pituitary gland, which is a miniscule droplet-shaped structure nestled deep within our heads at the base of the brain. For its tiny size the pituitary gland packs a mighty punch, pumping out hormones into the bloodstream that travel to distant receptors all over the body to regulate growth, blood pressure, energy management, the thyroid gland, the menstrual cycle, temperature, breastfeeding, water and salt balance … And, of course, labour. Basically, it keeps us alive. A colossal responsibility for something the size of a pea and weighing a featherlight half a gram.

Oxytocin floats around the mother's circulation until it tracks down and latches onto oxytocin receptors in the uterus. It's therefore a different type of hormone to prostaglandins that ripen the cervix; prostaglandins are made local to their target tissues and do not enter the bloodstream.

When the oxytocin receptor on the uterus is switched on by the oxytocin hormone, it gives an executive command to the machinery within the uterus that had laid dormant for years (if not its entire existence): to arouse and start contracting. It is fascinating that over the course of pregnancy the uterus prepares for labour by vastly upping the number of oxytocin receptors studded on its surface by a whopping 300-fold (that's 30,000 per cent). By the end of pregnancy, the uterus is heaving with battalions of oxytocin receptors – bolt upright, on constant alert, primed for active duty and awaiting the one auspicious day when a flotilla of oxytocin that has negotiated the stormy eddies of the circulatory system arrive from distant shores; a fleet of oxytocin created and unleashed by a benevolent pea-sized master that regulates the world but has only ever known utter darkness. They dock. And say, 'Lads and lasses, it's time'.

Oxytocin was discovered in 1909 by Sir Henry H. Dale. What is beyond weird – or pure genius – is that he isolated tiny bits of human pituitary that contained oxytocin and applied them to the isolated uterus from a pregnant cat. Just to see what would happen. What inspired the chap to contrive this oddball experiment – smearing snippets of human brain onto a womb freshly ripped from a recently purring feline – I couldn't begin to guess. But something dramatic happened: the cat uterus obligingly contracted. Using the Greek words 'quick' and 'birth', Henry named his discovery 'oxytocin'. Clearly, the name stuck. Forty-seven years after Dale's initial discovery, Vincent du Vigneaud synthesised pure oxytocin so it could be used medically, and he bagged a Nobel Prize for doing so.

To run the oxytocin through a drip, it's mixed into a bag containing a litre of sterile water and electrolytes (salt, potassium, calcium among other things). An infusion pump that sits on a metal pole next to the bed controls the flow rate, delivering exact volumes of the oxytocin mixed in the sterile water and electrolyte solution (Hartmann's solution is commonly used). The speed of the fluid flowing through the drip is related to the amount of oxytocin we are giving. Hence, running the Hartmann's and oxytocin mix at a rate of 20 millilitres per hour delivers half the amount of oxytocin compared to a rate of 40 millilitres per hour.

We steadily increase rate of fluid running through the drip over the course of hours until active labour kicks in. We are aiming for three to four strong contractions every 10 minutes, where each last around a minute. Pretty full-on stuff. Once active contractions are in full flight we stop increasing the rate, but we maintain the infusion speed at the same rate until birth. If we stop the trickle of oxytocin the contractions will usually peter out.

It takes roughly four to six hours from first starting the drip until we reach full strength contractions, but this varies enormously. The lead-up to active labour is usually much quicker for those who have birthed before.

Once contractions are at full strength, we manage labour much the same way we care for labours that start up spontaneously (which you will hear about very soon). It's just that we lent a hand to get things started.

Whether by acupuncture, a stretch and sweep, a balloon or prostin gel the cervix is now ripe, the uterus cocked and loaded. A few irregular contractions might have even appeared, teasing the nerves of the expectant mother and those around her.

We are now poised on the precipice of full-blown labour. Just like that nervy moment in the movie *Independence Day* when menacing spaceships hover over major cities with intentions undeclared; or when ginormous battalions of armed Orcs from evil Mordor stand in sinister silence at the walls of the mighty fortress Helm's Deep and we know an epic bloody battle will soon erupt; or when Meg Ryan makes first contact with the anonymous NY152 in an online chatroom in the 1990s romcom *You've Got Mail.* Tense stuff. I can barely watch.

In the next chapter, we release the slingshot and launch into full-blown active labour. Things could get hectic. So, take a breath. And read on.

Recap:
Gearing up for labour

1. The cervix is the opening of the uterus facing the birth canal. The cervix ripens as the time of labour draws nearer. Starting in the unripe state as a long, closed (and firm) tube, the cervix shapeshifts into a thin, stretchy, gaping hole, 2–3 centimetres open. Once transformed into this ripened state, the cervix is primed and ready for labour.

2. During cervical ripening, a mucous plug that was once wedged inside the cervical canal may topple out the vagina. Seeing the mucous plug – a stringy goop with the consistency of snot – does increase the chances that labour will soon fire up, but it's no sure sign that labour will spontaneously kick in.

3. There is quite a list of home remedies to kickstart spontaneous labour – guzzling castor oil, eating seriously spicy foods, sex, vigorous exercise and raspberry leaf tea. There is also acupuncture. Sadly, there is no firm evidence that any of them work. However, they are all very safe and women should feel free to give any of them a shot if they wish.

4. A stretch and sweep is where we place a gloved finger into the cervical canal and perform a few circular sweeps. There is evidence it is somewhat effective in starting up labour, but it's not a sure bet.

5. Induction of labour is a process where the clinical team gets labour going, instead of waiting for spontaneous (or 'natural') labour to happen. For those who need one, it is reassuring to know that there is strong medical evidence to show being induced does not increase the risk of medical interventions (such as caesars or instrumental births).

6. The first step to inducing labour is to ripen the cervix (only if it's unripe in the first place). Cervical ripening is achieved either by inserting a small balloon into the lower end of the uterus (where it sits just above the cervix and left in for up to 24 hours), or by placing hormonal preparations into the vagina. Cervical ripening is done a day before we get actual labour started.

7. The second step is to switch on active labour. This is done by breaking the waters (via an internal examination) then running the hormone oxytocin through an intravenous drip. Oxytocin directly stimulates the uterus to start contracting. Once the drip has started it can take around four to six hours to reach the full-strength contractions of active labour, but sometimes it can be a lot quicker.

Chapter 4

The waiting game: the first stage of labour

This is a critical chapter as most of the time spent in labour is during the first stage. Digesting what follows will demystify a lot of the 'goings-on' in the birth suite. So, let's leap right in.

If the first stage of labour adheres to nature's masterplan, then over some hours uterine contractions will edge the baby down the birth canal and the cervix will progressively dilate to 10 centimetres, or full dilatation. This then brings mum to the second stage – the next chapter of labour and of this book.

Two potholes can blemish the path to a smooth vaginal birth. Labour can stop progressing so that the cervix stops dilating. The second pothole is what's widely known as 'fetal distress', which is when the baby copes poorly with the stress of labour. Both are quite common and are the main culprits responsible for caesareans, which obviously short circuits the road to a vaginal birth.

Stalled progress of labour and fetal distress are the reasons why labouring women take an unplanned detour to the bright lights of the operating suite, so I cover them in quite some detail: why they happen, how we figure out they have happened, and our options if they happen. If either happen during labour, understanding them in advance will hopefully make the experience far less intimidating.

The first signs of labour

At the very beginning when the uterus starts contracting it's not painful. They commence as 'tightenings' – the uterus feels like it is squeezing and relaxing repeatedly. At first there are just a few per hour, and each lasts around 10–15 seconds.

Then over hours they build up in intensity, length and frequency. And, yep, at some point they become painful, though only mildly so at first. They are distinguished from pelvic or ligament pains by the fact that the epicentre of the pain is centred on the uterus (that big growth above the pubic bone that transformed the mum-to-be's walk into a waddle) and not lower down in the pelvis. Please remember this because many who are close to their due date and on high alert often wonder whether a heavy dragging pelvic pressure (like the baby's about to topple out) or sharp stabs knifing the vaginal region are labour. They aren't.

During this gradual build-up of contractions – the passive stage of labour – it's best to lie low at home. But it's the cue to dial the Batphone and alert the preselected support team. It's time for the spouse or partner to drag their butts back from golf day, no matter how smashing the day's scorecard is; and if the mum-to-be hankered for the comfort of her own mum fussing about her while labour builds up it's time to fire her a text (she was waiting for it anyway – her phone never strayed beyond arm's reach, even while on the toilet).

Many birth suites will invite women into the birth suite when the pains are coming and going every five minutes or so. This (almost always) provides a very safe margin to get to the birth suite in time.

While the contractions build up at home, mums-to-be can try out some of the simple pain relief measures described in Chapter

2 – a TENS machine if they had been sufficiently organised to acquire one, heat packs, a mollifying soak in a warm tub, standing in the shower under a soothing sprinkle of water – and they can take paracetamol. Some may wish to set the mood by burning an aromatherapy candle (any candle really, fake or real) or filling the room with music that suits their taste.

'Spurious labour' is an exasperating thing that befalls some pregnancies. This is where tightenings start up and continue for hours and hours, but they fail to ramp up and active labour doesn't kick in. The tightenings just plateau in strength and roll on, and on. And on. Without active labour kicking in, the cervix doesn't progressively dilate as it needs to.

Annoyingly, spurious labour can even stretch on for days; an exhausting state of sleepless limbo that can be terribly dispiriting. All birth suites have different policies for those who find themselves trapped in spurious labour and keep turning up to the birth suite, hopeful but unsure. Some will repeatedly send women home and ask them to patiently wait until active labour starts up (evidenced by a change in cervical dilation). And for some, this does happen, eventually. I think, if the poor mum-to-be looks utterly wrecked and had already presented to the birth suite at least once before, the kind thing to do is to offer an induction.

Spontaneously breaking the waters before labour starts

The 'waters' can break any time during labour; this is when the placental membranes spontaneously rupture and amniotic fluid gushes out. We call this 'ruptured membranes'.

In around a third of pregnancies, the membranes rupture before labour starts. Not sure why, but the sudden gush is often timed while women are dreamily luxuriating on ultra-absorbent white cloth couches. Or when sound asleep in bed where it artfully sidesteps an undersized mattress protector and seeps into an expensive mattress, finding itself a comfortable new abode. It's like it knows.

There is a high chance that after the membranes spontaneously rupture labour will promptly set in within hours. However, this is not for sure and some who rupture their membranes will be dismayed to find their uterus eerily silent on the matter hours or days later.

If mums-to-be discover they have ruptured their membranes, I suggest they give the birth suite a call. They are likely be invited in to be assessed. If the membranes have been confirmed as ruptured but labour is not setting in, an induction will be booked for some time over the coming days. We do this because once the membranes have gone there is a risk that opportunistic bugs (bacteria) could travel upwards through the vagina, through the freshly minted hole in the placental membranes, breach the amniotic cavity and basically have a bit of a party in the womb, rudely giving the baby a nasty infection. Therefore, it is a good idea not to leave women undelivered too long if they have ruptured their membranes and have reached 37 weeks gestation or beyond. We may hold off if a pregnancy is less than 37 weeks gestation and sit tight to give the preterm baby more time to develop in the womb. If we do this, an infection risk remains ever present so we need to monitor mum closely. We'd deliver regardless of gestational age if we suspect an infection is taking root.

Welcome to the birth suite

On arrival to the birth suite a midwife will greet the mum-to-be and a doctor will often pop by to say hello. All with warm, welcoming smiles (I know this because all midwives and doctors are friendly).

The mum-to-be and her selected support crew will be ushered to the room where she will give birth. Stepping into this special room can be an emotional thrill, as it makes it suddenly very real that baby will be arriving soon.

There will be a bed, one that bends in all sorts of directions. The foot of the bed can be reconfigured to accommodate stirrups if we need to place women into the lithotomy position during the second or third stage. The lithotomy position is where the mum lies on her back on the bed and legs are held in the air by padded holders (stirrups) that stick upwards from the end of the bed and sit under the calves. The legs are bent at the knees and the thighs rotated out. We place women in this position if we need to perform a forceps or vacuum birth, or we need to put in a few stitches to mend vaginal tears that have arisen while bubby was being born.

Some expectant women have a misplaced fear they will be left neglected in the birth suite room with no staff in sight for hours on end, huffing and puffing alone. This is not the case. Most birth suites allocate one midwife to exclusively care for one labouring woman. If the birth suite is busy, midwives are sometimes paired as teams of two to provide care for three labouring women. Therefore, highly skilled midwives will be spending a lot of time in the room with the labouring mum-to-be, providing attentive care, getting to know her and her support crew, and be on tap to answer questions. They will be a highly comforting presence.

Also, depending on the model of care, labouring women also get to know one of us too – the doctors on duty in the birth suite. We may meet the mum-to-be well before birth itself and we will visit regularly. Importantly, the doctors will work closely with the attending midwife and share management decisions. For some healthcare models such as private obstetric care, the mum-to-be may have already formed a close, trusting bond with the obstetrician over the months leading to birth (getting to know my own lovely private patients across their pregnancy – and to share more than a few laughs – is great fun). Also, there are some low-risk models of pregnancy care that are midwifery led (including private midwifery care). In these care models, the doctors may not pop into the room if the labour is progressing smoothly but are on tap to help should issues arise.

Many birth suites also have birthing balls or birthing stools that labouring women can try out. Most will also have an ensuite with shower or bath, so there is the option of warm water to help counter the pain in labour.

Women often wonder whether they can eat and drink during labour. They can, especially drinking. However, it's fair to say that most women are not feeling particularly peckish once in the throes of labour. Also, a borderline nausea can creep in for some women during active labour. So, by all means, pack some favourite snacks and drinks. However, I suggest simple things that do not sit too heavily in the stomach (perhaps not the time to launch into succulent, fatty barbeque ribs).

Also in the birth suite will be the cardiotocograph (CTG) machine which monitors the fetal heart rate. We are going to hear all about the CTG in rather a lot of detail shortly, so let us park it for now.

Finally, tucked into the corner of the birth suite room is a small setup to provide resuscitation for newborns who need it. There is usually a small mattress, a heat light that swings out over the mattress to radiate warmth on the newborn, and a few dials and knobs and tubing that can be hooked up to a small mask that helps support babies taking their first breaths. We will take a look at the resuscitation of babies that require it in the next chapter, but we first need to safely birth junior, so let's also set that one aside for now.

Monitoring the progress of labour: how slow is too slow?

During active labour each full-strength contraction should last around a minute to 90 seconds, with three or four occurring within each 10-minute period. It's pretty full on. But that's how strong and frequent contractions will need to be for the cervix to steadily dilate so that labour can reach the second stage.

To determine the strength of the contractions the midwife lays a skilled hand on the abdomen of the mum, directly on top of the uterus. The harder the uterus feels during the squeeze of the contractions the stronger we deem them to be. We grade the strength of the contractions as 'mild', 'moderate' or 'strong'; 'moderate' is of sufficient strength for us to declare someone is in active labour.

Once a woman is deemed to be in active labour, we perform vaginal examinations spaced around two to four hours apart to assess whether the cervix is dilating and labour is progressing. We are waiting for the cervix to be fully dilated (or 10 centimetres dilated). When this point is reached, no cervix can be felt whatsoever at the internal examination.

The average length of active labour is six to eight hours for a first-time mum, and often a fair bit shorter for a second-time mum. We doctors and midwives don't fuss when labour is progressing smoothly and the cervix is dilating, but we do when the rate of cervical dilatation is too slow or has entirely stalled.

So how slow is too slow? Whether a labour is induced or spontaneous, we judge the progress of active labour the same way: the rough rule of thumb is that once in active labour, cervical dilation should ideally be no slower than one centimetre per hour.

Let's say someone presents to the birth suite in active labour at 10 o'clock in the morning. If we perform an examination and the cervix is 3 centimetres dilated we may plan to reassess dilation again in four hours time, around 2 o'clock in the afternoon. By then we are expecting the cervix to have progressed to at least 7 centimetres dilatation. We then expect that it will be fully dilated at around 5 o'clock in the evening. If the labour is falling short of this pace of cervical dilation it captures our attention.

Why do we even bother keeping tabs on the speed of cervical dilation? Can't we just patiently wait? Stick in an epidural, and play Uno until the head pops out?

We pay a keen interest in the length of labour because excessively long labours can dangerously tire the unborn baby. I discussed in Chapter 1 how labour is taxing for the unborn baby because oxygen delivery reduces with each uterine contraction. Labour is a little like running a marathon for the unborn child and it's unsafe to stress junior in this way indefinitely (I can't quite believe I survived my own labour – I can barely jog 5 kilometres without feeling the ghostly chill of the grim reaper floating overhead and raining dribble down on me in hangry anticipation).

Stupidly long labours can risk becoming hazardous for the mum too. It can cause the uterine tissues to become waterlogged and friable. A little like soaking paper towelling with water, though nowhere as dramatic. This is a problem if a caesar is ultimately required at the end of a really long labour: the tired, fragile uterine muscle will bleed briskly during the operation, and it's more liable to tear in directions we don't want it to while we are getting the baby out. Occasionally, these tears are nasty and terribly difficult to repair (tears of the uterine wall continue to bleed until the edges are tightly sown together). All obstetricians will readily agree that performing caesarean sections after exhaustively long labours are far more challenging than those done for pregnancies that have only laboured a little while or not at all. However, if you are faced with a caesarean section after an epically long labour don't worry – we obstetricians are highly trained, and we can perform caesarean sections for all situations. We might just need to really concentrate and there may be less social gabbing on from us while we operate.

It is fascinating how the modern rules for defining speed of labour came to be – all based on a single study published by a Dr Friedman in 1955. The 1950s was an auspicious moment in history, one completely foreign to us. It was a time when the world was still licking its wounds from World War II, the Cold War had just started icing vast swathes of the globe, and miscreant youths were utterly hooked on the addictive properties of hula hoops. Telephone booth stuffing was a thing, where giggling college students piled as many of themselves into the booth as possible to break records (after all that effort, they presumably raced over to Big Al's Diner to slurp on strawberry thickshakes). Houses could be purchased for $7400. An era so foreign to us that people found *I Love Lucy* hysterical.

Friedman studied 1000 women who birthed at the Sloane Hospital for Women in New York, plotted the progress of cervical dilation on charts and published the average length of labour. On average it took first-time mothers 4.6 hours to go from 4 centimetres cervical dilatation to full dilatation (10 centimetres). He mathematically determined that cervical dilatation slower than 1 centimetre per hour was a sensible line in the sand to deem labour as progressing too slowly.

Held as the absolute truth for over 60 years, it is perhaps no exaggeration to say Friedman's 'one centimetre per hour rule' has guided the management of billions of births. And yet, the women he studied in the 1950s are almost nothing like most giving birth around the globe today. The New York cohort he studied were almost certainly all white, mostly in their 20s and a fair bit slimmer than many women of today (obesity slows labour). Weirdly, during the 1950s it was common practice to routinely sedate women during labour, something no-one does now (we hope).

Therefore, is this 'one centimetre per hour rule' at all relevant to labouring women of today?

Surprisingly, it wasn't until 2010 that the Friedman chart was seriously challenged. A consortium across the United States collated data from over 62,000 births from 19 medical centres and generated the Zhang chart. These were 'normal' pregnancies: defined as women who spontaneous laboured without being induced, had a vaginal birth and a baby that ended up being healthy.

The major difference between Zhang's chart to Friedman's is that it permits the definition of normal labour progression to be far slower. The average lengths of labour were similar in both cohorts; however, Zhang uncovered some very slow labours that ended up being successful vaginal births.

The enticing theoretical advantage in using the newer Zhang chart is that it permits a longer period of time for pregnancies to labour before we declare progress as too slow and need to then consider interventions such as caesars. It was hoped that using this new chart would drop rates of caesarean sections.

There is a lot of enthusiasm for the Zhang chart. The concept is very popular among those who are staunchly pro-vaginal birth and believe clinicians resort to offering caesars too soon during longer labours. Major obstetric societies in the US were early adopters and published official recommendations that the Zhang's chart should replace Friedman's (fun fact – I bought Professor Zhang a take-away coffee in Las Vegas).

Does using the Zhang chart actually decrease rates of caesarean sections? A major study in Norway tackled this question. It was a large clinical trial that ran across 14 birth suites – a major undertaking – where half used one chart and the remainder used the other. For enthusiasts of the Zhang charts the results were disappointing: there was absolutely no difference in the rates of caesars if the Zhang chart was used, compared to sticking with the '1 centimetre per hour' rule based on the Friedman Chart. Happily, baby health outcomes were the same in both groups.

Given there is no evidence that one is better than the other, I suggest labouring women trust the team managing their birth and let them define length of labour by following clinical protocols they are most familiar with. Regardless of which, the rough rule of thumb is that labour may be too slow if the cervix is dilating slower than 0.5-1 centimetre per hour during active labour. If this happens, we don't head straight for a caesar. There are some active management options we can try to get labour moving, which I will soon cover in this chapter.

Reasons why labour can slow down

There are a few reasons why labour progress slows or stops entirely, where cervical dilation does not change between vaginal examinations spaced over many hours.

Labour can stall when the contractions are too weak. They may not be strong enough, do not last long enough (they should last at least a minute) or are not frequent enough (ideally three to four within each 10-minute interval).

The second reason why labour progression may stall is a source of immense frustration – not just to obstetricians and midwives but also poor Alice in vignette two, whom we met in the Introduction. This is when the baby's head is in the birth canal but is facing the wrong way.

The best direction for babies to face is what's called the 'occipital anterior' position. Think of a fish swimming right way up out of a narrow cave. This is the occipital anterior position (the fish imagery only works if mum is on her back and the fish is swimming upright through the birth canal). In the case of a baby trying to squeeze its way through the birth canal, when in the occipital anterior position its mouth is closer to mum's anus, its eyes closer to mum's pubic bone. The baby is therefore facing mum's back.

The occipital anterior position offers the best chance of a vaginal birth because in this orientation, the shape of mum's pelvis will naturally flex the baby's neck, tucking the chin onto the chest. This presents the smallest possible head diameter that needs to squeeze through the snug birth canal. When the baby's head is fully flexed (chin on chest) what first emerges through the vaginal opening at birth is not the baby's eyes but the top of its head.

Labour can stall if the baby is in the occipital transverse position, where the 'fish' is heroically trying to swim sideways out of the cave. When a baby is in the occipital transverse position its mouth is close to one of mum's thighs and the eyeballs closer to the opposite thigh. This means one ear is close to mum's anus and the other ear just below her pubic bone.

The last position to note is the dreaded occipital posterior position, which is analogous to the fish attempting to swim through the cave flipped completely upside down. The baby's eyes are closest to mum's anus and the mouth just below the public bone. The baby's back is lined up adjacent to mum's spine and the baby is facing the roof.

Occipital transverse and occipital posterior positions are deeply infuriating reasons why labour progression can stall. We will still actively manage the labour and try to achieve a vaginal exit for baby, but when the mischievous little munchkin is in these positions – especially the occipital posterior position –

labour can be far slower, harder going and the risk that a caesarean section is the end result increases. These positions mainly stall the labours of first-time mums; very often someone who has birthed before will spontaneously swivel the baby to the more convivial occipital anterior (upright fish position) as labour progresses.

We figure out the direction babies are facing during the same vaginal examination done to determine cervical dilatation. We feel for patterns in the grooves running along the surface of the baby's head – called suture lines – that correspond to the front, top and back of the head. Suture lines are the borders between bones that make up the skull. After birth, the suture lines completely fuse, so don't bother groping about the top of your own head as you won't find them. For additional clues as to which direction bubby is facing, we can also try to feel where his ears are. Sometimes when we are still unsure, we can check the position of the baby using a trusty ultrasound which we wheel into the birthing room.

The third reason why labour can stall is that the baby is simply too big, what's called macrosomia. Why don't we save women all the bother of going through a failed attempt at a vaginal birth by doing an ultrasound during pregnancy to find all those with macrosomia and offering them a caesar straight up? It's because even though we can suspect the baby is large in utero, we can never be sure it is indeed big until it's born and plonked on the scales. It may come as a surprise, but ultrasound is not absolutely precise in determining fetal size – it can miss quite a few, as well as falsely label others as macrosomic. Furthermore, some women can comfortably birth babies just over 4 kilograms as they are blessed with pelvises that are unduly accommodating, while others will struggle with smaller babies. We simply cannot predict who will – and will not – succeed in having a vaginal birth without giving labour a shot.

The last reason why labour stalls is because mum's bony pelvis, or her pelvic tissues, are too narrow for the baby, a condition called cephalopelvic disproportion. I realise a lot of mums worry about this, especially those who are slight in build and chanced upon love with a gentle giant. But be reassured that cephalopelvic disproportion is less common than many people think. It is also not possible to tell whether a pelvis is too small to accommodate the passage of a baby unless the mum gives labour a shot. In the past, clinicians have used X-rays and CT scans to measure the width of the bony pelvis before labour, thinking this could predict who may be headed for trouble. But we now know these tests are hopeless in predicting whether a labour will stop progressing because the pelvis is too small. They do little more than zap the unborn baby with X-rays it doesn't need and these tests shouldn't be ordered for this reason.

The options if labour has stopped progressing

If we suspect labour is advancing too slowly – contractions not strong enough, baby not facing the right way, baby too big, or pelvis too small – we usually follow the same playbook to cajole the cervix to resume dilating again. Remember that during the first stage the singular aim is to reach full dilatation – 10 centimetres wide – so that the second stage of labour can commence.

If the membranes have not ruptured yet, we will break them (see Chapter 3). Breaking the waters can be enough to stir up the uterus to contract more strongly, which gets the cervix dilating again, especially for those who have birthed vaginally before. After breaking the waters, we wait a few hours to see whether stronger contractions indeed kick in or not.

If rupturing the membranes has no effect, or they were already ruptured, the only option left is to start running an oxytocin drip (again see the section on inducing labour in Chapter 3). The aim is to increase the rate of the oxytocin drip until the uterine contractions are at full strength: three to four strong contractions within every 10-minute interval, where each contraction lasts a minute to 90 seconds. We do not want them to happen any more frequently or last any longer than this or we risk tiring the baby (remember oxygen flow to junior reduces during each contraction so we need to strike a balance). Starting the oxytocin drip is obviously only an option for spontaneous labours that have stalled, not labours that were induced in the first place as they will already have oxytocin running.

It does not matter what we suspect may be the underlying cause for labour stalling, we will usually still offer the oxytocin drip. This is because we can't truly know the reason, or reasons, why labour has stopped progressing. Also, whatever the underlying reason, we can't be sure that the oxytocin drip can't overcome the problem. For instance, we won't know whether the baby is really too big for mum's pelvis unless we give the oxytocin drip a shot.

Using oxytocin is more likely to end in a successful vaginal birth if the baby is occipital anterior, but it is still worth giving it a go if it's not: those in non-occipital anterior position can still edge to full cervical dilation with the help of oxytocin. Once fully dilated (the second stage of labour) there may be an option for us to help turn the baby the right direction using forceps or the ventouse (vacuum) – more on this in Chapter 7. Even better, sometimes we score big time where stronger contractions that kick in with the oxytocin drip magically swivels the baby to an occipital anterior position over the ensuing hours (such happiness when this happens).

Ultimately, the oxytocin drip is the last roll of the die. If the cervix still flatly refuses to dilate after many hours of the oxytocin drip (variously called 'obstructed labour', 'arrested labour', or 'failure to progress') the only remaining option is a caesar. Although we can do caesars very safely (see Chapter 8), we know for many it is plan B and not the birth outcome they had hoped for when they first stepped into the birth suite earlier in the day. But we need to get baby out somehow.

Labour is a risky time for the unborn fetus

Now we have covered the problem of obstructed labour let's turn our attention to the other major reason why labour in the first stage ends in a caesarean section birth. It's what's widely known as 'fetal distress' and is when we suspect the fetus may be in peril because of dangerously low levels of oxygen.

How risky is it for a baby trying to be born? Being a natural event crafted over eons by mother nature, surely all babies plop out safe, sound and squawking? Many people believe this – some stridently – but it's just not the case.

In the 1980s, Ronald A Howard of Stanford University devised a scoring system called the 'micromort' to compare the relative riskiness of different activities. Micromort stands for 'micro-mortality', where one micromort equates to one in a million risk of death. Skydiving, for instance, scores 10 micromorts per jump, riding a motorbike incurs one micromort per 9.7 kilometres (a pretty precise calculation right there) and each hit of heroin risks 30 micromorts (don't do it, boys and girls!). Walking 30 kilometres scores one micromort; running the exact same distance ups the risk to seven micromorts. (Which is what I – a wannabe runner with the lung capacity of a meerkat – have long suspected: running is seven times more deadly than walking.)

A research team later calculated the number of micromorts incurred by babies on the day they are trying to be born. They landed on the rather unsettling conclusion that the day you are trying to be born is the riskiest day of your life. In fact, you'll never face the same daily risk of death until you are 92 years old.

For babies trying to be born in the United Kingdom the risk of dying during childbirth is a weighty 430 micromorts (430 in a million risk). And for babies attempting to be born in the United States the risk lifts to 1460 micromorts. If you happen to be a uterine occupant during labour in South Africa your risk of dying rockets up to a horrific 8200 micromorts (19 times higher than the UK). Climbing Everest scores 37,932 micromorts, which means scaling the highest mountain in the world is only 4.6 riskier than a baby in South Africa striving to make it out of mum's womb alive just to become part of the world. Trying to be born is a risky undertaking.

Why is labour so dangerous for the baby?

To supply oxygen to the fetus, mum's blood vessels thread through an intricate lattice of muscle fibres of the uterus to reach the placenta. There, at the microscopic border between the maternal blood and placental surface, is a miraculous exchange vital to life. Oxygen leaves mum's blood, crosses to the placenta and is loaded onto fetal blood. Flushed with oxygen, the fetal blood flows through the baby's circulation to distribute the precious gas across the body. The oxygen is voraciously consumed to generate energy, keeping the trillions of cells in the body energised and in a general state of contentment.

In turn, the waste product carbon dioxide diffuses the opposite direction, back through the placenta into the maternal bloodstream, to be carted off to the mum's lungs and harmlessly breathed out (hopefully next to a nice tree with healthy green leaves). Refer back to Chapter 1 for more on the great job the placenta does.

During labour this system is put under stress. With each contraction the uterus squeezes into a tight ball which squishes the maternal blood vessels coursing through it. This slows maternal blood flow and oxygen delivery to the placenta and fetus. So as labour chugs on the amount of total oxygen the fetus receives progressively falls and at some point, this really strains the baby. At the start of labour, we cannot predict which babies will cope well with this strain and which will struggle.

Therefore, babies need their backs watched during labour. If there are strong suggestions that an unborn baby is imperilled by critically low levels of oxygen, we can save it by performing a caesarean section. Once removed from a hostile environment and safely out in the world, it is no longer buffeted by waves of reduced oxygen flow caused by caused by uterine contractions. Instead, it switches to its own lungs to draw breath and can freely suck in all the oxygen it needs.

Watching for fetal distress

Fetal heart rate patterns can detect dangerously low oxygen levels in unborn babies. It appears some sort of arcane, mystic art. The clinical team in the birth suite peers at the fetal heart rate patterns being spat out of a machine called the cardiotocograph (known as a CTG) and can somehow divine whether the baby has plentiful access to oxygen or may be suffocating and hurtling towards strife. How is it even possible to glean levels of fetal oxygen by observing fetal heart rate patterns?

The brain has a ferocious appetite for energy and devours crazy amounts of it just to keep going. Oxygen is consumed in all cells – especially those in the brain – to manufacture gazillions upon gazillions of microscopic energy powerpacks called ATP. The packets of ATP energy then power the 30+ trillions cells that makes us 'us'. As I am sure you know, in the body: oxygen = energy = life.

It is an interesting fact that the newborn brain hogs 65 per cent of the body's total energy needs. Presumably the brain of a soon-to-be born baby also gobbles up a similar lion's share of total energy.

Given its insatiable thirst for energy ('feed me…feed me…') the brain is one of the first organs to feel it when oxygen supplies run low – such as when the unborn baby is under siege from decreased oxygen flow caused by uterine contractions.

So as strange as it sounds, we use fetal heart rate patterns as a fancy sensor that detects low oxygen delivery to the brain. The brain is constantly micromanaging fetal heart rate patterns and when starved of oxygen, the stressed neural circuits alter the signals it transmits to the heart. This changes the fetal heart rate patterns, and the doctors and midwives can see them in real time on the cardiotocograph readout (we then infer if the brain is low in oxygen, it is likely the rest of the baby isn't getting the life preserving oxygen it craves either)

Monitoring the fetal heart rate with the cardiotocograph

Two sensors from the CTG machine are strapped onto mum's belly. One detects the fetal heart rate and the other senses when uterine contractions are happening.

An ultrasound sensor continuously records the fetal heart rate at every moment (beats per minute), similar to the heart rate readout on a Fitbit or Apple Watch. The fetal heart rate pattern appears as a squiggly line scrawled on a very long piece of paper continuously spat out from the CTG machine, or on a computer screen (in more eco-friendly birth suites). CTG machines also have audio so the fetal heart rate can be heard as well.

The second CTG sensor detects when contractions are happening. This readout appears as a line that runs in parallel below the fetal heart rate. Each contraction looks like a narrow hill where the crest of the hill is timed with the peak of the contraction when the uterus is squeezing at its most tight. The width of the 'hill' corresponds with the duration of the contraction whereas the height approximately equates with how strong it is.

Sometimes we are unable to maintain a reliable continuous readout of the fetal heart rate, no matter how much we fiddle with the placement of the ultrasound sensor on mum's belly. If this happens, we can perform a vaginal examination and place a small clip directly on the fetal head, called a fetal scalp electrode.

It is placed on any part of the fetal head that's poking through the partially dilated cervix.

The very end of the fetal scalp electrode is a tiny spiral needle twisted into the skin of the fetal scalp (but very superficially, just a few millimetres deep). The electrode continues as a thin electronic wire that runs along the length of the vagina, emerges out of the vaginal opening and runs to the CTG machine. It measures electrical impulses rather than sound waves and is a more direct way of monitoring the fetal heart rate then the ultrasound sensor strapped on the belly. Once in place, we can remove the ultrasound fetal heart sensor from the belly, but the second strap holding the sensor detecting when uterine contractions are happening is left on.

How we interpret the fetal heart rate patterns from the CTG

This section gives you a little insight into how we make sense of fetal heart rate patterns. I added it thinking some may find it fascinating. But you don't have to remember any of this – we won't be asking the mum-to-be or the support team what they think of the CTG heart rate patterns (I'd be a bit worried about the expertise of those in birth suites that do). So, if this section is doing your head in, feel free to skip over to the next section.

The fetal heart sets a cracking pace with a resting heart rate – what we call the baseline rate – tapping away between 110 to 160 beats per minute. This is way faster than in adults and we only reach such speeds when engaging in strenuous activities such as running (for those foolhardy to take on the 7 micromort risk).

There are some fetal heart rate patterns that are highly reassuring when seen on the CTG tracing as they only appear when the fetal brain has a plentiful supply of oxygen to snack on. One is a periodic rise and fall of the fetal heart rate above the baseline. They look like little hills that rise above the baseline rate then descend back to baseline. We call these 'reactivity' or 'accelerations'. They often disappear from the CTG tracing as labour advances, but don't worry if they do – their absence does not mean the baby is low in oxygen.

The second reassuring feature we like to see in the fetal heart rate trace is constant squiggling: fast 'up and down' dynamic fluctuations in the fetal heart rate that dance about the baseline rate (a little like the earthquake Richter scale readings captured on a seismograph that we see in big budget Hollywood disaster movies). These arise from constant small adjustments in the fetal heart rate coordinated from a well-oxygenated brain (why the brain bothers expending the energy to perform such precise second-by-second micromanaging is beyond me). This pattern is called 'variability' and is rated 'normal', 'reduced' or 'absent'.

Normal variability is a good sign as its presence suggests the baby is well oxygenated. We deem the CTG readout as having normal variability if the fetal heart rate speed is bouncing up and down the baseline rate with an amplitude of 6–25 beats (looks like: /\/\/\/\/\/\/\). 'Reduced variability' has a lesser amplitude (less 'up and down' compared to 'normal' variability), whereas with 'absent variability', the CTG fetal baseline pattern is almost a smooth line (--------). Reduced variability puts us on alert and absent variability can make us edgy, as low fetal oxygen levels can certainly cause this.

What also makes us wary are periodic dips in the fetal heart rate below the baseline called 'decelerations'. They appear as upside down hills (or simply dips) on the CTG fetal heart rate tracing and they catch our attention because they can also reflect low fetal oxygen levels. However, it is important to keep in mind that the presence of decelerations does not always mean fetal oxygen levels are low. There are different types, where some are more worrying than others. And some types are not particularly concerning at all.

Lastly, we get a bit toey if we see the baseline fetal heart rate rising up and up and sailing north of 160 beats per minute. And staying above 160. We call this a fetal 'tachycardia' and it classically appears when labour has dragged on for a really long time. It's what befell poor Alice in vignette two, back in the Introduction. One cause of such an inexorable rise of the fetal heart rate baseline is, once again, low fetal oxygenation levels, although it isn't the only cause.

How accurate is the CTG?

The CTG is a good diagnostic test but it isn't perfect. Its great strength is that it's a 'sensitive' clinical test. This means it's great at detecting babies suffering from low oxygen and rarely misses any. So, if the CTG readout is normal, we can be pretty certain the baby is fine. And that's a good thing.

The problem with the CTG is that it is not a 'specific' clinical test. This means if the test is abnormal the fetus *may* be suffering from low oxygen but it's not for sure. The test can therefore overcall, sometimes incorrectly flagging babies as being stifled by low oxygen when they weren't, and, in fact, were doing just fine. It is not hard to understand why: as mentioned above, the presence of non-reassuring fetal heart rate patterns (such as decelerations) may or may not mean there are low fetal oxygen levels. The CTG simply reports these patterns and the clinical staff is left to decipher which babies are truly struggling.

It's not complete guesswork, though – far from it. It is perhaps best to think of the CTG test like a traffic light system. If the CTG is normal we get a green light which says the baby is fine. And we have already established that we can believe a green light – if the CTG says the baby is okay, it is. A green light can be trusted and means it's super safe to continue labour.

At the other extreme we occasionally see fetal heart rate patterns that are really bad news, an unambiguous 'red light' signal. When present, there is a high probability the baby is in critical danger and a prompt caesarean section will likely be lifesaving (or delivery expedited by forceps, or vacuum, if the cervix is fully dilated and the baby is low enough in the birth canal). A red light signal accurately picks babies who are truly distressed: if seen, everyone would agree urgent delivery is what's needed.

But the picture can get murky when the CTG throws up fetal heart rate patterns we might classify as 'amber' signals. When they appear, it is likely the baby is stressed but it can be difficult to figure out just how badly. If we return to the marathon analogy, if we see an amber signal the baby could be a little breathless but coping fine, or it may be really struggling and in danger of falling short of the finishing line. Sometimes it can be really hard to know.

Unfortunately, in the birth suite we grapple with ambiguous 'amber signals' pretty often (there are in fact shades of amber – some are more worrying than others, but none are a sure bet of anything). Watching *possibly* concerning CTG patterns that run on for hours upon hours can really frazzle the nerves of doctors and midwives given the stakes are so high. It is therefore understandable that clinicians will recommend a caesarean at some point just to be on the safe side, but the baby may have coped okay with more hours of labour. I would quickly note that a caesar isn't harmful for the baby (and overall, a safe operation for the mother) but the opportunity for a vaginal birth is lost.

In a nutshell, the big benefit of using CTGs is that they are great at identifying unborn babies with low oxygen levels. I have little doubt its use has saved countless babies. But its drawback is that it can lead to caesarean sections and forceps births that were not essential.

Not perfect, but until we find something more accurate to pick low fetal oxygenation the CTG remains our best tool to spot babies teetering at the ledge of a mortal precipice – at risk because of perilously low oxygen supplies caused by labour. And in urgent need of saving.

Things we can do to improve concerning CTG fetal heart rate patterns

When the CTG shows an 'amber' or 'red' signal there are a few things we can try to get more blood and oxygen flowing to the unborn babe. If they succeed, it will improve the fetal heart rate patterns.

Firstly, if there is an oxytocin drip running, we can decrease the amount being given (or stop the infusion entirely) to lessen the strength and frequency of the contractions. This gives the baby a rest, a chance to catch its breath. Once the CTG fetal heart rate patterns improve we can increase the rate of the oxytocin drip again to strengthen the contractions, and we just hope that bubby copes better the second-time around.

We can also change the position of the mother. If the mother is lying in bed, we can ask her to roll onto her side. This helps because when the mum-to-be is flat on her back, the uterus can squish onto major blood vessels that are underneath and running along the top of her hard, bony spine. This compromises mum's blood supply to the uterus, placenta and fetus. A roll to one side can flop the uterus off these important vessels, improving blood flow to the unborn babe.

We can also increase the rate of the sterile fluid running through the drip as increasing the total volume of mum's circulation can improve the delivery of blood and oxygen to junior.

If we see fetal heart rate patterns that are really worrying, we can inject powerful drugs (such as salbutamol or terbutaline) that act rapidly and temporarily to stop the uterine contractions for around 20 or so minutes. Ceasing the contractions gives the babe a chance to draw breath.

Fetal scalp blood sampling

If the CTG fetal heart rate pattern is throwing up an infuriating 'amber signal' and we are unsure about the true oxygen levels in the baby, some clinicians will perform what's called fetal scalp blood sampling. This can provide further information about the unborn baby's oxygen status that doesn't rely on fetal heart rate patterns.

When fetuses have suffered from really low oxygen levels for a long time something ominous happens. Sensing they aren't getting the oxygen they need to make energy, cells throughout the body switch to another way of generating power. A temporary way to make life-preserving energy that does not need oxygen. It's just like a back-up generator that kicks in when the lights go out.

This alternate way to make energy when there is not enough oxygen comes under the fancy name of 'anaerobic metabolism'. It is a rapid response survival switch to keep cells alive but is a far less efficient way to make energy compared to consuming oxygen.

The problem with anaerobic metabolism is that it generates lactic acid as a nasty by-product. This lactic acid percolates out of cells and enters the fetal bloodstream, making the blood more acid and lowering the pH. Like a sinister poison, the acid spreads throughout the body and leaches into organs. The fetal brain is particularly sensitive to acidity and can sustain hefty damage that can be permanent. Not good.

Thus, anaerobic metabolism kicks in during emergencies as a rapid response, back-up generator to keep energy supplies flowing for a while until oxygen levels are restored, but it can't be the way we generate energy indefinitely because acid build up is an unfortunate by-product (if we could safely depend on anaerobic metabolism to indefinitely to make energy in place of oxygen, we wouldn't need to breathe in oxygen at all. We could probably manage a casual stroll along the ocean floor, spooking startled marine wildlife).

Fetal scalp blood sampling is a procedure where we obtain a few drops of the fetal blood by lightly scratching the unborn baby's scalp and measuring the pH levels of the blood (low is bad), or levels of lactic acid itself (high is bad). If pH or lactic acid levels in the fetal blood are normal then we can be reasonably certain that oxygen levels in the baby are okay at the moment, and that labour can safely continue.

To perform fetal scalp blood sampling, we place a cone through the vagina where the narrow edge of the cone is placed flush on the unborn fetal head that is poking through the partially dilated cervix (the cone is little like the hollow cardboard cylinder in the middle of paper towelling except one side is wider than the other). The cone protects mum's vaginal skin by holding it out of the way. Using a tiny blade at the end of a long plastic stick that's inserted through the middle of the cone, we make a small scratch on the scalp of the unborn baby's head. We collect a teeny drop of blood that wells up at the scratch and analyse it in a very sensitive machine. If we find that the pH of the fetal blood sample is low, or that lactate levels are high we can be more certain the baby is indeed suffering from low oxygen levels and we can proceed to a caesar with greater confidence that we have made the right call.

There are some limitations. As you might imagine, fetal scalp sampling is fiddly to perform. And it only provides a snapshot of lactic acid levels at the time it is done; we don't get continuous live updates like we do from a CTG. So if we get a comforting result from fetal scalp sampling that's great, but if the CTG pattern further deteriorates we cannot remain reassured.

Fetal scalp sampling is only sporadically performed. Many birth suites do not perform it. It's hardly done in the United

States. Its supporters will enthuse that for the right situations it can prevent some caesars by providing reassurance in situations where the CTG is ambiguous, and clinician is mulling over whether it would be safer to offer a sunroof escape for the baby.

Intermittent monitoring instead of the CTG

We do not always go straight for the CTG to monitor the fetal heart rate for every labour. For pregnancies assessed as low risk we may perform 'intermittent monitoring' instead. To do this we use the same hand-held Doppler device deployed to audibly listen to the fetal heart at each antenatal visit – the little machine that makes the whooshing sound with each heartbeat.

Every 15 minutes the midwife listens to the fetal heart rate during, and just after a contraction. We are listening out for decelerations, the transient slowing of the heart rate speed that we've just heard all about. If decelerations are heard (the sound of the fetal heart rate slowing down and speeding up again is very familiar to us) then we move to CTG monitoring for the rest of the labour. If no decelerations are heard, we can continue with intermittent monitoring.

We go straight for continuous monitoring using the CTG for pregnancies that are higher risk, if an epidural is inserted and for all labours that are induced.

Meconium liquor: another sign of fetal distress

When stressed, some unborn babies do a small poo inside the uterus, what we call meconium. Sounds just wrong but don't worry – it's very different to the unspeakably putrid nasties we manufacture as adults (especially after a delectable fat laden feast). Meconium is sterile, not smelly and not even brown. But it does stain the amniotic fluid and turns it from being straw-coloured to a shade of green. This charming mix trickles out of the vagina and seeing it appear is how we discover meconium is present. We call this cocktail blend 'meconium liquor'.

Meconium liquor is graded by sight as thin or thick. Thin meconium has a light green hue, like diluted green cordial; thick meconium is darker green and can even have lumpy bits. At times thick meconium liquor takes on the uncanny appearance of pea soup and we affectionately call this 'pea soup meconium' (delicious).

The presence of meconium is another sign that the fetus could be low in oxygen and stressed. But it's no sure sign that the fetus is in trouble and many with meconium liquor are just fine. The presence of meconium perhaps sits in the bucket of an 'amber signal' on a CTG. Thick meconium liquor is believed to have a stronger link with fetal distress than thin.

Seeing meconium alone doesn't mean we need to deliver the baby immediately. But it is useful to know, as we add this snippet of information to the overall clinical picture to guide decision-making. For example, let's say we have been sweating over a CTG with an 'amber signal'. The sudden appearance of thick meconium liquor may be the trigger to recommend a caesar as the safest path. Alternatively, if meconium is seen in a second-time mum who is otherwise dilating rapidly, we may sit tight and let the labour continue, as we can anticipate a vaginal birth will happen soon.

A final thought – trust the team caring for you

I wish to leave you with some really important points about the whole business of fetal distress and interpreting the CTG.

First, bear in mind that the presence of decelerations (transient dips in the fetal heart rate) does not always mean fetal oxygen levels are low. So don't panic if you see the fetal heart rate periodically dropping during labour because it is common where often, fetal oxygen levels are just fine. Please let the doctors and midwives interpret the CTG fetal heart rate patterns.

Secondly, fetal heart rate patterns are not considered in isolation but used to help paint a clinical picture. Dramatically different management decisions can arise from an identical CTG tracing, depending on the clinical scenario. Let's say we encounter an identical CTG fetal heart rate pattern in two different labours, a pattern that sits in the 'amber' zone. One of these cases is a first-time mum who is only 4 centimetres dilated with an occipital posterior baby, already noted to be dilating slowly (slow progress between two vaginal examinations spaced many hours apart) and a trickle of thick meconium liquor appears. The clinical picture suggests we are a long way off from birth and if the labour is left to continue the already stressed baby is very likely to face the hazard of many more hours of reduced oxygen supply. Overall, none of this scenario bodes well for the prospect of a safe vaginal birth and a sensible decision may be to offer a caesar. In contrast, if the exact same CTG pattern is seen in a third time mum with a history of fast labours and she has already rocketed along to 8 centimetres dilated within an hour or two, it is probably safe to let labour continue as we can anticipate birth is around the corner (meaning the baby won't endure many more hours of further stress arising from labour).

So, my point is that interpreting the CTG is a skilled art where doctors and midwives integrate information from fetal heart rate patterns with the clinical situation. And we only become expert at using fetal heart rate monitoring to make sensible clinical management decisions after spending years in the birth suite providing care for hundreds of pregnancies.

Therefore, I do urge all mums to trust the team providing care on the big day.

I am sorry that this was a rather chunky chapter. Well done for making it through to the end (I barely did myself).

However, the first stage of labour is 'core business' and really deserved a good going over. I hope the read has well and truly erased much of the mystery of the birth suite. I've given a description of the birthing room, and explained that the mum-to-be will get a midwife caring for them who will be spending a lot of time in the birthing room. And I discussed how we monitor the progress of labour, reasons why labour might stall and our options to get things moving if it does. I also described how we monitor the baby to keep the precious little tot safe.

And it is my strong hope that these insights will empower mums and make the experience in the birth suite during the long first stage of labour less scary. Even interesting. Possibly rewarding.

In the next chapter, we will move on from core business to the business end. Birth.

Recap: The first stage of labour

1. In around a third of pregnancies, the membranes rupture before uterine contractions start. If this happens there is a high chance labour will set in within hours although it's not for sure. If contractions do not set in after spontaneous membrane rupture women may be offered an induction to kickstart labour over coming days.

2. The first stage of labour – where the cervix progressively dilates to 10 centimetres open – is divided into the passive and active stages. The passive stage starts from when contractions first appear from nothing and gradually build-up but are yet to be in full flight. This can last a variable number of hours. Most birth suites will suggest women go through passive stage at home, but they should feel free to keep in contact with their clinical team.

3. During active labour there are around three to four contractions within every 10-minute time period, where each last about a minute. The active stage lasts six to eight hours (although there is enormous variability) and the cervix is steadily dilating. We assess the rate of cervical dilatation by regular vaginal examinations spaced every four or so hours. Sometimes they are done more frequently.

4. Most will spend active labour in the birth suite, cared for by a highly skilled midwife. She can adopt any position, can eat

and drink, stand under a shower, modify the ambience with the room (music, candles, aromatherapy, dimmed lighting), and select from an array pain relief options we covered in chapter three.

5. There are a number of reasons why the labour progress can stall (where the rate of cervical dilatation is either slower than 0.5-1 centimetre dilatation per hour, or dilatation has stopped all together). These include the contractions being too weak, the baby is too big, is facing the wrong direction ('occipital anterior' is the best direction for bubby to face); or mum's pelvis is too narrow to let the baby through.

6. If labour stalls, options to get it moving again are to break the waters (if they aren't already broken) or run an oxytocin drip intravenously (if one is not already running). If these fail to get the cervix dilating, the only option left is a caesar.

7. Active labour can be a risky time for the baby because with each squeeze of the uterus during contractions there is reduced oxygen delivery to the placenta, and to the unborn bubby. Many babies cope just fine with this stress, but some will struggle. A small number do not cope at all and are in danger of falling off the edge if they are not rescued with a timely caesar.

8. To identify babies that may be suffering from concerningly low oxygen levels, doctors and midwives monitor fetal heart rate patterns during labour. They will use either a

hand-held Doppler device to listen to the fetal heart rate at regular intervals, or they will apply the cardiotocograph which continuously monitors the fetal heart rate. If there are strong suspicions that the unborn baby is in serious danger than a caesarean section may be recommended to keep the baby safe.

Chapter 5

Time to push: the second stage of labour and vaginal birth

I am not sure whether you have seen a goat give birth. It's an impressively slick 'no fuss' affair. The only sign that the doe is in labour is a subtle change in its personality. As if it has bad guts (like what we might acquire after overindulging in a fatty goat curry).

During labour, the doe may sway a little, bleat in annoyance at the inconvenience, breathe a little heavier or grind its teeth. Then sure enough, the kids plop out one by one, closely followed by the placenta. The kids then scramble onto their feet, prance up to mummy and start sucking. The doe then deals with the ravenous hunger generated from being in labour by chowing down on the placenta and wolfing down the lot. And that's it. (By the way, for only $29 Australian dollars (+ GST) anyone can purchase 60 goat placenta tablets for their nutritional needs. Apparently from certified New Zealand goats, which sounds top quality to me.)

In contrast, as we have discussed at length (complete with my mind-bending fish swimming analogy), human babies trying to be born can get stuck. Or find themselves suffocating from the effort. And we will later hear that these risks persist throughout the second stage – right up until the baby is out.

So why on earth do our furry, bleating friends find childbirth so easy while we humans find it challenging? Eons ago when we were slimy slugs dreamily paddling about in shallow, tropical ponds we were faced with a choice. We could evolve much like the rest of the animal kingdom – acquire the skills to bound across grassy plains at speed on four legs and affectionately greet one another by licking faces with long agile tongues – or stand up on two legs and develop the faculties to greet each other by waving (no closer than 1.5 metres and only after two squirts of hand sanitiser manufactured with >70 per cent alcohol) and speaking (or mumbling 'hello' through a three-layered cloth mask). By opting for the two-legged evolutionary option our pelvises narrowed in diameter, as this is apparently biomechanically more suited to bipedalism. But this narrowing of our bony pelvis has unfortunately made it more of a tight squeeze for babies to venture from point A (womb) to B (outside world).

Just to spice things up and make childbirth even more challenging, we made another sensible evolutionary decision – to become smart and acquire bigger brains. To accommodate the expanding bulge of neurons our heads simply got bigger.

Bigger head. Smaller pelvis. Not a clever combo, and that's why we don't spit out babies with the nonchalant ease that goats do. But take heart: we do birth a fair bit less smoothly, but we do have some significant survival advantages over a goat. Such as being less sumptuous in a delicately spiced curry.

While we have established labour can sometimes be a bit of a slog for humans, the fact we have reached this chapter means we've at least negotiated the first stage. Exciting, we have reached full cervical dilatation and within a few hours – and within the hour for some – the long-awaited cutie-pie will be born. So let's stop musing over how smooth birth could have been had we instead evolved to stride about on all fours, possessed udders, spiky horns, knittable fur or nifty egg laying abilities. Let's return to being human and hear about the final steps how our precious (albeit large headed) babies are born. Happily, there aren't too steps many left – we wait a little, do some spirited pushing and baby emerges. Childbirth is then over.

In this chapter, as well as birth itself, we will touch on a few other things.

Once freshly arrived in the world, the baby can take a little while to fire up its lungs (recall they lie dormant while baby is in the womb). Therefore, when junior first appears they may spook the parents by looking a little blue, a little floppy, and needing a little emergency resuscitation. We will take a look at resuscitation by the bedside so it's not so frightening if required for the birth you are involved in.

When the baby's head makes its final exit through the vaginal opening it can cause some tearing. And sometimes, we deliberately make a small cut at the vaginal opening while the head is passing through, called an episiotomy. We'll cover episiotomies and vaginal tears.

There is also an uncommon emergency called shoulder dystocia where the baby's head emerges but the shoulders remain stuck in the womb. We will cover how we deal with this occasional predicament.

But first, let's start by hearing about how the baby takes its final journal through the birth passage and how long it takes if it runs to plan.

Waiting before pushing

It is an exhilarating milestone. After many hours in the first stage of labour, the midwife has just done another internal examination, formed a smile and made the call. Mum has arrived at full cervical dilatation. No cervix to be felt whatsoever.

On hearing this the almost-mum may be immediately psyching herself up to push with the very next contraction. I therefore warn you ahead of time that once full dilatation is reached many clinicians suggest waiting an hour or so before pushing. This is what's known as the 'passive' second stage of labour.

The reason we suggest holding off immediate pushing is that even though the cervix may be fully open there may still be some distance between the baby's head and the outside world. Therefore, it makes sense to give some time for the head to descend down the birth canal under the steam of continuing contractions before mum starts active pushing. The hope is that this will shorten the starting distance between baby and the outside world when pushing begins. By doing this, it may increase the chances of a vaginal birth.

Also, although pushing is hard work for mum it is also strenuous for the baby – it decreases oxygen delivery to the baby and is liable to prompt fetal heart rate patterns on the CTG to deteriorate. Therefore, doing everything we can to minimise the length of time actively pushing is a good strategy in case the baby does not take nicely to the strain.

However, any time there is a feeling of an unbearable urge to push – a sensation triggered by the baby's head being really low in the pelvis and tantalisingly close to the outside world – we suggest women wait no longer and just get on with pushing. The head is low enough.

Not all clinicians suggest waiting before pushing. Some believe it adds nothing but time (research studies have not uncovered clear evidence supporting the concept of waiting. In fact, some studies have puzzled us by reporting it offers no benefit). I am an enthusiast for a little patience and giving passive stage a good hour or so before pushing commences.

Pushing

This really is the business end of labour. If giving birth were a movie this would be the final scene. Rightly, mum holds centre stage and everyone else crowds about her – the invited support team, midwife and the doctor.

We touched upon the technique of pushing in Chapter 1. During each push, the labouring mum fills her lungs to 60–80 per cent capacity. And pushes hard, with all they've got. Full throttle. Claret face, eyes widened, bulging veins, 'head-about-to-burst' type pushing.

With each contraction, where each lasts a minute to ninety seconds, mums can usually fit in three consecutive pushes (or even a fourth). Each sustained push continues for an effortful 10-15 seconds (meaning during every minute long contraction, three of these pushes are done in quick succession). This means the almost-mum only gets about a minute's respite between contractions to catch her breath from the effort of pushing. Hardly anything, but something. Active second stage can be pretty taxing.

My firm message to support persons reading this book is this: please, step up to the plate. The spirits of the person you are supporting can flag when she has pushed for a while but doesn't sense the baby is budging. Exhausted, she can feel trapped in a lonely place. Here is where your task is so important – steadfast encouragement and emotional support will be of inestimable help. Just a few choice words, timed well: 'good work', 'you can do it' sort of thing. Be on tap to offer sips of water. An affectionate wipe of the brow. Warm, loving eye contact to say you are with her.

Even with an epidural running, many can still feel when the contractions are happening, sensed as a painless squeeze of the uterus. If so, this is very useful as it can guide mum when to push. For those with a dense epidural block and unable to feel contractions don't worry, the midwife can lay a gentle hand on the belly and direct mum when to push. I have seen plenty of women push out their baby with an epidural running.

I acknowledge that active coaching and 'three pushes per contraction' is very common practice, but some birth suites advocate no coaching and letting women do whatever their bodies tell them. I have no handle on how successful this freeform approach is, and if it works for some then I am all for it. I think it makes a lot of sense to push at the same time as uterine contractions are happening because the mum is (literally) combining forces with the power of the uterus. And, of course, I have seen stacks and stacks of successful births with this common-sense approach.

How long the period of active pushing lasts before baby emerges varies immensely. It's usually around half to a full hour for a first-time mum, but it can even drag on for two or so hours (for those in the US, it seems widespread practice to let pushing run into a third hour). Conversely, for some really lucky mums the baby pops out really quickly, even within the space of a few contractions (if you are a first-time mum and this happens for you, it is a monumental win as it doesn't occur very often).

Happily, for second-time mums the length of time spent actively pushing before baby emerges is usually a whole heap shorter. And for very experienced mums, such as those having their third or fourth babies, just a few pushes may be all that's needed. I recall a pleasant memory where a lovely private patient of mine having her third baby leisurely waited for full dilatation while watching the Australian Rules Football grand final on TV in the birth suite (clearly she had an epidural in). During the third quarter I gently informed her it was time to push (tactfully timed during a quieter moment in the game, so as not to spoil her viewing pleasure). And asked whether we ought to switch off the TV. She considered it for a second and casually blurted out 'nah' (I knew her well; we had bonded over three pregnancies). So we went with her unconventional birth plan – watching the AFL grand final live during active pushing. Just a few pushes (suspiciously timed during commercial breaks) and the baby popped out. It was such a nice birth. I wish births were all so easy, where all the drama remained boxed in the TV and not in the birth suite. But I will note she earnt this right – her first birth was nowhere near so simple.

Positions for pushing

Women can push in many positions – they don't have to be lounging in bed, unless they have an epidural running, as their legs may be too wobbly to take on other positions. Women can push standing (advocates enthuse that this enlists the aid of gravity), squatting, on all fours on the ground (on a mat), or kneeling with the upper body upright and the arms resting on the side of the bed, and even walking.

Most, however, are content to push while on the bed, with their upper body semi-up right. They may find it helpful to adopt what's called a semi-lithotomy position, where the feet are placed on footrests on either side of the bed, as this opens up mum's pelvis. Pushing in bed but but lying on one side is another position some women find comfortable.

The highly skilled midwife attending the birth can provide suggestions and accommodate whatever pushing position best suits the mum-to-be. But should mum settle on more exotic positioning, please spare a thought for the amazing midwife who is charged with constantly checking whether a head is peaking through (especially important if mum is standing as we do not want bub's entry into the world announced as a head-first clunk onto solid hospital flooring), monitoring the uterine contractions, keeping tabs on the fetal heart rate and documenting events as they happen. It's a lot to do and they need to be pretty flexible (and supple) if the mother elects to push squatting, standing or walking.

Crowning: when the head emerges

A thrilling moment. I have witnessed many vaginal births, but my spirits still lift when the long-awaited head is finally seen jutting out of the vaginal opening. Particularly after watching the mum gallantly push for a long spell with grit and resolve.

The short period while the baby's head is tenting open the vaginal opening is called crowning. At this stage we are tantalisingly close to having a baby freshly born.

Crowning is like watching someone push their head through a thick, turtleneck jumper. At first, just a slither of head is seen in the distance. More and more of the head then emerges, which tightly stretches open the entire perimeter of the head hole. Finally, the head pops right through.

There are a few things to bear in mind during crowning. Firstly, the stretch of the vaginal opening causes an unpleasant sensation of extreme burning on the skin (not felt if there is an epidural on board). It is unavoidable and little can be done other than to encourage women to push through this. They can look forward to the horrid burning feeling dissipating rapidly once the baby is out.

Secondly, when a decent amount of head is poking through the vaginal opening we ask women to stop full-throttle pushing. They need to slow it down to controlled, stop-start pushing, guided by their midwife or obstetrician. We do this so that the widest diameter of the head eases through the vaginal opening nice and slowly, which protects mum's tissues and minimises tearing (think of an adolescent jamming their head through that tight turtleneck jumper with force, compared to someone slowly easing their head through a beloved jumper they had personally knitted).

Other things we may try to decrease the risk of tearing during crowning is placing a moist warm towel on the perineum as the head emerges (the skin area between the vaginal opening and the anus, which is the region most prone to tearing); or applying pressure on baby's head to keep it flexed (tucking the head down onto the chest, as this minimises the diameter of head required to squeeze through the vaginal opening). These tricks are part of the instinctive art of the experienced midwife, obstetrician or primary care physician assisting the birthing process.

We may also perform what is called an episiotomy. Once a fair proportion of the head is poking through and the vaginal opening is terrifically stretched, we place scissors at the lower edge of the opening and make an incision a few centimetres long. The cut is angled sideways towards the thigh, and slightly downwards. If an epidural is not in, we will first inject local anaesthetic to numb the area before performing the episiotomy.

Episiotomies are done to protect the anal sphincter, the important muscle that rings the opening of the anus and is the gate that controls bowel function. Vaginal tears happen more frequently than we would all like – the consequence of birthing babies endowed with rather sizeable craniums. I am afraid tears are very common for first-time mums: most will sustain some sort of tear rather than escape without one. An episiotomy is an attempt to prevent spontaneous tears that run down the perineal skin to the anus and rip the delicate anal sphincter muscle.

The direction of the episiotomy is therefore deliberately angled away from the anus in the hope it will provide a vaginal opening that is spacious enough to let the baby pass and leaves the anal sphincter intact.

If we perform an episiotomy, or a tear happens, they are repaired straight after birth and most of them heal quickly with excellent results. We will take a closer look at tears, episiotomies and how we mend them in the next chapter.

Luckily, mums who have had vaginal births before acquire accommodating and stretchy vaginal outlets. This means second-time mothers who have birthed vaginally already (or have had a prior forceps, or vacuum birth) often sustain no tearing. Often, they won't even need an episiotomy. And if tearing happens for a second-time mum, it is usually very minor and easily mended.

The moment – birth of the baby

If the tale laid out in this book could claim a climactic scene, it's now. An emotion-charged event prepared for over many meandering months. And for some, a moment with an emotion-charged lead-in spanning years, pinpricked by halting beginnings. An event that seemed so far from reach even earlier in the day when mum first tentatively stepped into the birth suite.

Birth itself.

With a few final pushes the head emerges, usually with the baby facing towards the anus – the 'occipital anterior' position. Once the head is birthed, the midwife or doctor will gently reach in with a finger and probe the baby's neck to see whether there is a loop of umbilical cord around it. If there is, we simply loop it over the head to loosen it. It is therefore no big deal if the cord is around the neck: contrary to the imagination of many, babies do not suffocate themselves at birth by having their umbilical cord pulling progressively tighter around their necks like a terrible noose (and for the tiny number that try, monitoring fetal heart rate patterns will alert us to problems early and we can intervene).

While sticking out of the vaginal opening, the baby's head will then swivel 90 degrees to the left or right, so that bub ends up facing one of the maternal thighs (a process called restitution). The doctor or midwife may manually guide this process. Once the head has restituted, mum is asked to give a final push and the shoulders and body slips out in one slick motion.

The baby is then born.

The newborn

We will place the precious bundle onto mum's tummy and chest, straight into her longing arms. It may come as a shock how wet and slippery the new bundle of cuteness is. The skin will likely be coated with a glistening sheen of amniotic fluid which may be faintly tinged with green if there was meconium liquor.

Often, bubs will be adorned with white waxy goo called vernix. It is slopped all over the skin of the unborn (and just born) baby, providing a patchy underlay to the wet amniotic fluid. Vernix is probably sludge sloughed off the fetal skin during its time in the womb and though theories abound, we really don't know whether it serves a purpose. Unsurprisingly, chemists at leading cosmetic companies have strived to mimic vernix as a skin cream, presumably so that adults can transform their aged, sun-ravaged integument into the smooth suppleness that covers a newborn. I have my doubts as to whether such overpriced lotions contain the requisite magical properties to pull off a Benjamin Button.

Babies lose heat very quickly once out of the warm environment of the womb. The midwife will therefore wipe off the wet slop covering the baby. The baby can then be left skin-to-skin with mum, commencing the miraculous road of mother–child bonding (a loving journey lasting decades – until an older version of mummy summons the courage to delicately enquire when the 'baby' intends to leave home – given they have just turned 34 and draw a healthy income, but are still manifestly incapable of operating the front loader).

Once the baby is out, the emotional ambience in the birthing room vastly transforms. The tense anticipation that had mounted for hours melts away into a collective sense of relief. After a fleeting moment of disbelief that it's finally all over, everyone is talking freely – happy chatter. The atmosphere morphs to being chilled and relaxed. Eyes reddened, tears, wide smiles all round. Laughs. It's nice.

I have been delivering babies for 20 years and still feel elated when seeing a new being join the world with a bewildered cry. And yes, as the obstetrician responsible I still feel a pang of relief. A great moment.

Resuscitating the baby

For months the baby's lungs lay dormant, its oxygen-absorbing role admirably performed by the placenta. A child's first few breaths is a complex marvel of human physiology where blood vessels bypassing the lungs rapidly clamp shut (to be forever closed) as the lungs fire up. This often happens the instant baby appears but for some, the lungs hesitate before starting up. If there is a delay before breathing establishes the baby can emerge a little blue, floppy and in need of resuscitation.

If a newborn emerges floppy and does not promptly pink up, start to breathe or cry, we will take the baby over to the resuscitation area (or we may wheel in a portable resuscitation cot). Although midwives and obstetric doctors are skilled in basic neonatal resuscitation, we may invite an expert paediatrician to come help. They are specialists in babies and children – we affectionately call them 'baby doctors'.

If the baby worked hard during labour and was getting less oxygen than it would have liked while in utero (where perhaps the CTG heart rate pattern was an 'amber' signal – or even 'red') then the chances of requiring resuscitation are higher.

We do a few things to get the baby breathing. We begin with simple measures such as warming the baby by wiping off the goo on the skin, providing warmth via a heat lamp (which usually sits overhead), and giving bub a vigorous rub using cloth towels which provides tactile stimulation (we don't smack the baby, that's so 1950s). These steps are often sufficient so that within a minute after the birth, the baby will blurt out a belated cry, and get on with the job of breathing and pinking up. We then quickly return the little sugarplum to mummy.

If we find baby's heart rate is lower than 100 beats per minute (it should be between 120–160) then we will place a little mask over the mouth and nose which delivers short bursts of air directly into the airways (called 'continuous positive airways pressure'). There's nothing scary about this mask – it's similar to the ones that some adults wear whenever they sleep to overcome house-shattering snoring caused by their upper airways collapsing (a condition called obstructive sleep apnoea – the mask not only makes them healthier, but also their marriage). During resuscitation, the newborn may only need the mask for mere minutes.

A very small number of babies remain floppy even after all these steps. Also, their heart rate may remain slower than normal, and they may still not be breathing. If so, we will proceed to chest compressions. Also, we may need to intubate them – place a tube down the windpipe to support breathing.

If more involved resuscitation steps are required – chest compressions or intubation – then once we stabilise the baby we will move her to the neonatal special care nursery (or neonatal intensive care) for closer monitoring. If this happens for the birth you are involved in, be reassured that the outcomes are usually excellent. For most babies, the stay in the nursery is brief and they are returned to their parents within days. During their time in the nursery, parents can visit their baby for as long as they like. And depending on how bub is doing, they can hold and cuddle their little tot.

The message here is that after birth, a brief delay in establishing breathing and minor resuscitation steps is not uncommon. It happens, and quite a number of mums (plus spouses, birth partners and support people) will witness such an event; the baby can't be dumped straight onto mum's tummy but instead is whisked over to the resuscitation area. Don't be alarmed if it occurs. Just know from the outset it is rare for babies needing resuscitation to do terribly. In most cases the visit to the resuscitation area is a brief one and the baby is returned straight back to mum's arms in the room within minutes. So, if it happens, please let the clinical team do what they are highly skilled at. And trust them.

Cutting the umbilical cord

Let's return to the lovely scene of the newborn perched on mum's tummy being fawned over by those around him. At this point the long umbilical cord is still attached to junior's navel. It runs through the vaginal opening, along the vaginal canal into the cervix and plugs into the placenta, still inside the uterus.

The cord needs cutting. The midwife or doctor will place two clamps across the umbilical cord a few centimetres apart which blocks off the blood flow (if left unclamped, blood will spurt out of the cut edge – a messy scenario best avoided).

We offer the partner scissors to cut the umbilical cord (in between the clamps). Cutting the cord feels like cutting through cooked calamari. Some partners are too squeamish to cut the cord and we fully respect this (no, not a wuss at all – their birth partner just went through an epic nine months and gave birth, but cutting the cord is just a bit much…). If they opt out, we can do it.

Lights, camera, action in the birth suite

Cutting the cord is a photo opportunity. I therefore hope the partner or spouse had the foresight to bring a phone or camera. (They are in deep trouble if they haven't. Such a lapse is almost as heinous a crime as the best man or woman misplacing the wedding ring.) One of the thrills of my job is to switch roles from obstetrician to cameraman: I relish the opportunity. I might even say (immodestly) that I have a pretty decent eye. The photos I take are similar to those of dignitaries lined up to officially open a refurbished community centre (or some other over-budgeted, tax-funded public construction), where a VIP holds oversized scissors poised to cut a red ribbon and everyone grins broadly at the cameras snapping away. I get the support team to do a similar pose, but it's surgical scissors hovering over an umbilical cord, not red ceremonial fabric. After the still shot, I then flick the smartphone setting to video and record the actual (ceremonial) snip of the cord. All the while, I am diligently censuring what's in frame to ensure the photos and movies can be safely shared (no, I don't do weddings, sorry. But thanks for asking).

It has been fascinating to see how practices have evolved over two decades. When I first started delivering babies, I would see a clunky camera looped around the partner's neck. Nowadays it is just a smartphone, whipped out of a back pocket. However, I note with keen fascination that on occasion, a support person will bring in a camera. If they do, it's no longer one of those compact 7 mega-pixel devices of circa 2007 (those useless little machines with an infuriating time delay of half a second between pressing the camera button and the grainy low-res shot being actually captured). Instead, it's usually a meaty beast. A whopper. I have even noticed the odd times where the birth partner (evidently a camera enthusiast) wields an intimidatingly big camera with an enormous zoom about the length of the baby's leg and the diameter of a bread plate. The type of professional camera one might use to capture distant celestial bodies. I'm sure there's a good reason and I'm just too simple to understand why such a huge apparatus is required to capture shots of one's baby cooing a mere 30 centimetres away. Though I do not doubt the pictures captured will be crisp, sharp and of top quality.

You may have heard about delayed cord clamping and be attracted to its touted benefits. This is where we wait a minute or two before we clamp the umbilical cord, then sever it. There are two theoretical benefits. First, it may allow more time for blood to run from the placenta to the baby, filling up its circulation with more blood before permanent separation. Another theory is that delaying cord clamping can facilitate the transition to breathing which reduces the risk for resuscitation.

Large studies have been done that show that delayed cord clamping holds some significant health benefits if the baby is very preterm. However, if the baby is at an advanced gestation the jury is still out that a delay in cutting the umbilical cord is useful. My hunch is that for most babies at full term, delayed cord clamping may not offer huge health benefits as most are already robust and will do well anyway (though I would also add that studies are ongoing on the possible benefits of delayed cord clamping for babies at full term. Some excellent researchers are convinced it is useful and some paediatric societies officially recommend it. The new mum can either request delayed cord clamping or simply go with what's common practice in the birth suite providing care for the birth).

Shoulder dystocia

Sometimes we have trouble delivering the shoulders after the head has popped out, a situation called shoulder dystocia. The baby's 'anterior shoulder' – the shoulder just behind mum's pubic bone – is wedged stuck behind this bridge of bone. It needs to slide under it for the baby to get out. It's uncommon – occurring in 1–2 per cent of all pregnancies – but it can be quite an emergency.

Shoulder dystocia is a time-critical emergency because once the baby's head is out, oxygen levels drop acutely as if it is breath holding. We have around five or so minutes to deliver the rest of bub.

If it happens, things can get dramatic for a short while with jolting suddenness. The midwife or doctor in the room will request urgent help. An emergency code may be announced through overhead hospital speakers (at our hospital, obstetric emergencies are a 'code pink'). Very quickly, other staff members will stream into the room to render assistance.

All this sudden flurry of activity can be distinctly unsettling. But please don't be alarmed as the extra reinforcements have come to help and we have done this together many times before.

We perform some specific manoeuvres to deliver the baby when the shoulders are stuck. For example, with mum on her back, clinicians on both sides of the bed will hold mum's legs, bend the hips and knees fully, and rotate the hips outwards to open up the pelvis. Another set of hands will push on mum's lower tummy just above the pubic bone, applying direct pressure on the unborn baby's anterior shoulder to slide it under mum's pubic bone to free baby. At the same time, another one of us will be directly facing the vaginal outlet, holding the head or reaching in to hold onto the upper body, and trying to deliver the baby. In most cases of shoulder dystocia, these steps will fix the problem and the baby will safely exit mum within a minute or two of the emergency being called.

In more severe cases of shoulder dystocia, the baby stubbornly refuses to budge with these steps. We will then precede to more advanced manoeuvres. For instance, we may reach into the uterus to locate and deliver the posterior arm through the vaginal outlet – the arm belonging to the shoulder closer to the anus. Once we manage to pull out this arm the rest of the baby will slide out.

If we have spent a number of minutes trying to deliver baby because of a shoulder dystocia, it may arrive quite flat and in need of resuscitation. Luckily, we can call another code to quickly summon paediatric doctors to help (in our hospital, we call this a 'paediatric code blue').

Rarely, shoulder dystocia can go pretty badly, where the baby emerges in poor shape and needs some heavy-duty resuscitation efforts. This is most uncommon and if it happens, most will still fully recover.

Thankfully, most cases of shoulder dystocia are a short-lived drama – over in a minute when the baby tumbles out in good health. The code is then stood down and all the extra helpers file out. The room quietens again, and the serenity returns.

We've made it. Over the last few chapters we have walked through the steps culminating in a vaginal birth. Plan A for most. A hearty congratulations.

Dotted along the journey were a few moments of excitement: dodgy CTG fetal heart rate patterns, a slow labour needing the oxytocin drip, a minor episode of shoulder dystocia, a little resuscitation. But we got there, and the baby is well. Indeed cooing, and so cute as to be near edible.

Thus far, we have stepped along the path to a vaginal birth. I might just gently remind you that the spectres of fetal distress and the labour failing to progress hover right up until the moment of birth. In the chapters following the next, we will hear about plan B exits: forceps, vacuum and caesarean sections. These are our bail-out options when it is apparent that a vaginal birth is not going to happen, or is too risky to wait for.

However, even for a vaginal birth, it's not quite over. If you recall, there is another stage of labour. Mercifully, the third stage of labour is far shorter than the previous stages but on occasion, also packed with drama. Only when this final stage is done and dusted can the clinical team leave the new family in peace (though I can't promise the newborn will – they are fond of making full use of their newly inflated lungs). The final stage of labour will be covered in the next chapter.

Recap: **The second stage of labour and birth**

1. Women arrive at the second stage when they reach full cervical dilatation. Like the first, the second stage is often split into a passive stage (where we encourage women not to push just yet, for an hour or so) and active stage (which is when full-throttled pushing happens). Some clinicians bypass the passive stage and get women pushing as soon as it's apparent that the second stage is reached.
2. The pushing stage is often done within an hour but can last longer. There is enormous variability how long it takes to push out a baby – for some really lucky ones, the pushing stage is over in a matter of minutes. Pushing is generally far shorter for those who have birthed a baby via the vagina before (even if by forceps or ventouse).
3. Pushing is a strenuous undertaking. A common approach is to push during contractions. Women are asked to give an almighty, sustained push for 10–15 seconds, quickly snatch their breath and immediately perform another push of the same duration. Then do it again a third time. Women can usually fit in about three pushes with each contraction (because each contraction is typically 60–90 seconds in length). Between contractions, women can rest.

4. Women can adopt a variety of positions while pushing, from sitting semi-upright in bed, squatting, kneeling (perhaps with arms resting on the side of the bed), on all fours and even standing.

5. The time when the baby's head is visible and tenting the vaginal opening is called 'crowning'. If there is no epidural, crowning can cause a rather intense burning sensation on the skin surrounding the vaginal opening. Happily, this 'set alight' unpleasantness promptly dissipates soon after the baby is born.

6. As the baby emerges through the vagina, we may perform an episiotomy, a small cut at the opening of the vagina. An episiotomy is done to encourage any tearing to angle away from the anus (and particularly the anal sphincter, which is the important ring of muscle that gives us bowel control). If an episiotomy is done or there are vaginal tears, we will mend them immediately after the birth.

7. Once out, the newborn sometimes takes a little time before drawing in its first breath. If this happens the baby might need a short period of resuscitation. This is not uncommon and is usually over within minutes whereupon the babe is promptly handed to mum for hugs. Also, its often just light resuscitation where all is needed is some breathing support (the need for chest compressions is far less common). Please do not be alarmed if resuscitation is needed for the birth you are involved in as outcomes are nearly always good.

8. Uncommonly, the head is born but the shoulders of the baby are still stuck inside the womb, a situation called shoulder dystocia. It can precipitate a short-lived moment of drama where assistance is summoned, helpers rush into the room and the clinical team performs few specific manoeuvres to get the baby out. If this happens, please trust the team. And be reassured that almost every time, the baby is birthed within minutes and is perfectly fine.
9. The end of the second stage heralds the arrival of a special bundle of joy. At long last. Congratulations.

Chapter 6

Tying up loose ends: the third stage of labour

Finally. The baby is out. Is it all over? Are we there yet? Sadly, we can't abruptly end proceedings in an instant, like movies can with a definitive roll of credits. The difference between us and the shiny and bright characters on the silver screen is that we are buffeted by the realities of life. They aren't.

Heroes entertaining us on the big screen – whether they be a melodically inclined Austrian family trekking along scenic mountain peaks having just escaped Nazis by hiding in a spooky monastery, or a heroine saving the universe from evil grandpops who smirks while spraying forth lightning from gnarled fingertips to destroy spacecraft – do not seem inconvenienced by mundane matters that plague real people, such as mortgage repayments, fender benders or hauling luggage about (I note Rey wasn't carting about scratched Samsonite suitcases stuffed with spare Jedi garb). And they never seem troubled by gripey attacks of bowel cramps or messy gastro (imagine if John Wick had to simultaneously grapple with the perilous consequence of being decreed 'excommunicado' from the world of assassins and explosive diarrhoea).

Mired in reality, we need to do something our fictional friends don't. Tidy up. And yes, after the birth there is a bit of tidying up to do.

For starters, in all the excitement it might have escaped your notice that the placenta is still inside the womb, patiently waiting. That needs to come out. There may be tears or an episiotomy and they'll need mending. Heavy bleeding trickling out the vagina can happen soon after the birth – a postpartum haemorrhage. If it does, it'll need swift action to stem the flow.

Here we will walk through some bits and pieces that may need tidying up during the final stage of labour. Then for those who have a vaginal birth, their journey ends here.

Delivering the placenta

Many pages ago I proposed that the placenta doesn't receive the accolades, love and attention it richly deserves. It gave us life: placentas now long gone once supported you, me, our grumpy neighbour, their grumpy neighbour. Grumpy in-laws. The cat. It is criminal that the pathetic, worm-like appendix gets far more airplay. That mischievous slug does nothing useful, never supported a life (except gut bugs and maybe a worm) and has anti-social tendencies to become a kamikaze nuisance by trans-mutating into a super-sized ball of pus threatening to pop.

But now the baby is out, the placenta's role-sustaining life is over. And I am sad to say it is time for it to leave. Though let us not forget to wave a fond farewell with moistened eyes (as we slide its goopy carcass into a yellow 'biohazard' bag to face a fiery destiny of some 800+ degrees, as per the local health act).

Once the uterus has been emptied of the baby it naturally contracts – this is called involution. As the uterus squeezes into a tight ball the placenta shears off from the inner lining and is released, or 'separates'.

Soon after the birth we administer a dose of oxytocin which actively contracts the uterus and aids placental separation. The oxytocin injection reduces the risk of severe bleeding and is given into the thigh, or via an intravenous drip directly into the circulation.

To ease out the placenta from inside the uterus we perform what's called controlled cord traction. The midwife or doctor will place one hand across the lower abdomen to feel where the uterus is while the other gently pulls on the umbilical cord segment still dangling outside the vagina. The placenta then neatly slides out.

Happily, this step – officially the third stage – usually does not take long. For most pregnancies the placenta is out within 10–15 minutes after the arrival of the new miniature person.

Manual removal of placenta

In roughly 2–3 per cent of births the placenta fails to separate from the uterus, what's called a 'retained placenta'. We patiently wait an hour for the placenta to emerge before making the call that the placenta is properly stuck.

Unfortunately, we can only sort this out by taking mum for a brief visit to the operating theatre. We need to make a move to theatre quite promptly because while the placenta remains stuck inside the womb there is a risk that at any moment, torrential bleeding starts up. Nice to avoid.

Under the cover of a short general anaesthetic or a spinal anaesthetic (we add more drug into an epidural if one is in place), we obstetric doctors perform what's called a 'manual removal of placenta'. We don a really long sterile glove (I mean long: the sleeve ends at our elbows). We reach into the uterus via the vaginal opening and birth canal. Shaping our hand flat like a spatula, we dislodge the placenta off the wall of the uterus. Just like sliding a spatula under a pancake to lift it off the frying pan (though we need to work a little harder to sheer the placenta off the womb). Emptied of its overstaying houseguest, the uterus can finally contract down unimpeded. And if there are vaginal tears that need mending, we'll fix those while we are in theatre.

We can manage retained placentas safely, but it's a nuisance. Mum has just conquered childbirth and wants to be left in peace to cuddle the new addition to the family. Instead, we pass the baby to the spouse or partner, and whisk her off to the operating suite for an otherwise quick procedure.

Retained placentas sure are annoying things.

Vaginal tears and episiotomies

May I introduce you to a marvellous structure that endows us with the luxury of controlling our bowels and bladder – skills that, I am sure you'd agree, we are all rather fond of? This unsung hero keeping us dry, clean and decent is called the pelvic floor. It's the same muscle that's actively squeezed by those who remember to do their pelvic floor exercises (community message – if you manage to get into a lifelong habit of doing these otherwise mundane exercises your twilight years will be drier).

It is not easy to visualise where this hidden structure sits but let's give it a try. The pelvic floor is a muscular sheet made up of overlapping muscles that form one structure. They are attached along the inner walls of the bony pelvis. From there, the pelvic floor muscle sweeps down inside the pelvic cavity towards the vaginal outlet and ends by surrounding the rectum (the terminal end of the bowels) and sitting under the bladder, giving support to both. It also integrates into what's called the perineal body, which is a nub of fibrous tissue in the perineum (the segment of tissue between the lower opening of the vagina and the anus).

I appreciate I might have lost a few of you (sorry, but it's like putting down in words how to tie a shoelace). Can I test out this analogy to see whether it helps you better picture the pelvic floor? Imagine an empty ovoid sports stadium, with angled stadium seating (like, for instance, most cricket and soccer grounds). That's the approximate shape of the bony pelvis. During childbirth a (rather gigantic) baby falls head-first from the sky, through the middle of the stadium and through a massive hole in the grassy sports ground itself. Now, drape two thirds of the empty stadium seating with a seriously enormous sheet of muscle – this seating area represents the bony attachment of the pelvic floor muscle to the pelvis. Imagine this muscle (obviously an intimidating whopper) sweeps down – nice and taut – and inserts along the edges of the grassy sports ground on the opposite side of the stadium seating where the muscle originates. Lastly, picture (an epically big) bladder resting on top of this sheet of muscle. Immediately behind the bladder is a hole where the (also alarmingly huge) rectum plunges through.

If I have utterly lost you, don't worry. It's not important to picture where this retiring sheet of muscles sits within the pelvis. I do wish to convey the point that this sheet of muscle plays a key role keeping us continent.

And being so close to the action it's in the firing line during childbirth.

I mentioned in the previous chapter that as the baby's head emerges there may be some tearing, or we may perform an episiotomy. Tearing can arise anywhere around the vaginal outlet and the skin adjacent to it. Tearing also often involves the muscular layer beneath, which is none other than the pelvic floor muscle (for those who actually followed the stadium analogy, tears of the pelvic floor most commonly involve the section of muscle that inserts along the edges of the grassy sports stadium). Because we are often repairing tears in the pelvic floor muscle itself (as well as the overlying skin), it's important we do a good job of repairing vaginal tears.

We grade tears according to their severity. A first-degree tear only involves skin; either the vaginal skin (wrinkly skin inside the vagina) or the skin on the surface surrounding the vaginal outlet. A first-degree tear may also involve some of the superficial tissues just below the surface of the skin, but the pelvic muscle remains intact. In contrast, it is classed as a second-degree tear if there is also tearing of the muscle.

First and second-degree tears are common. In fact, first-time mums are far more likely to sustain some sort of tear or an episiotomy than escape without either. I would quickly add that nearly all of them can be mended with rapid recovery and excellent outcomes.

Third-degree tears are a little more serious. The injury is similar to a second-degree tear, but the anal sphincter is also torn. With a width of about 3 centimetres, this important structure circumferentially surrounds the opening of the anus and is the muscle we can voluntarily squeeze at will and gives us bowel (and flatal) control. Many of us may be too shy to utter its name (though we are at times tempted to accuse administrators with an abiding love of red tape of being one), but we can all agree it is a pretty important friend. It literally does all the sh**ty work for us. It's the anal sphincter we are trying to protect if we perform an episiotomy.

Overall rates of third-degree tears in the birth suites run at around 3–5 per cent of vaginal births for first-time mums having a normal vaginal birth, meaning they are not altogether rare. They happen more often for forceps or vacuum births (around 5–10 per cent). Conversely, they occur far less commonly for those who have had a vaginal birth before. A third-degree injury can be a partial tear through the sphincter, or a full thickness tear. When they happen, expert repair is obviously required.

Episiotomies may involve the underlying muscle. So, for the purposes of repairs, episiotomies are usually equivalent to a first, or second degree tear.

Mending perineal tears or episiotomies

To mend vaginal tears, we position women in the lithotomy position – lying on their backs (their upper bodies semi-upright so they can hold her precious newborn), legs held up in the air with padded holders (stirrups) that sit just under the calves, and the thighs rotated outwards. The doctor or midwife performing the repair sits in front of the vaginal outlet, directly facing the tear.

During the repair, mum can certainly continue cuddling and focussing on her gorgeous newborn. In fact, we encourage it – a lovely distraction.

We firstly inject local anaesthetic into the area to numb the tissues. This isn't needed if there is an epidural running.

We then sew up the layers. Almost all tears or episiotomies involve a split in the vaginal skin and this is mended using a continuous running stitch. Next, if there is injury to the muscles of the pelvic floor – a second-degree tear – we bring the edges together by placing a series of stitches. Finally, we close the skin where we often use a technique that nicely buries the suture material out of sight so when the job is done, no stitches are visible.

Happily, the stitch material dissolves by itself and does not need to be removed. The new mum should freely take painkillers as needed, enough so that she can comfortably move about. The pain usually settles quickly to a background nuisance within days and most will be pain free after a week.

If there is a third-degree tear we often repair these in the operating theatre. Yes, it is a hassle to move mum to theatre, but operating theatres are far better set up to undertake more complex surgical tasks then the birth suite. In theatre we carefully identify the ends of the anal sphincter and suture them together. Then we proceed with the rest of the repair, like how we just described.

If we have repaired the anal sphincter, we may prescribe antibiotics for a few days (an infection during healing of this delicate muscle is best avoided) and laxatives to keep the bowels moving smoothly, so mum avoids straining while the anal sphincter muscle is healing. During the first few weeks after the repair some women may be distressed by a few unsettling episodes of partial loss of bowel control (or control feels a little lax), but with the passage of time such symptoms will improve for most.

I will just mention in passing that there is something called a fourth-degree tear. This is a tear that not only involves the sphincter but also the delicate wall of the actual rectum – the tube that transports poo. This is pretty serious and most definitely needs expert repair in theatre. Happily, it is also very rare: I have only seen one in my two-decades career, and entire careers will only encounter a handful. And after it is mended well it can recover completely.

Most tears heal promptly with excellent results. In fact, the perineal region heals remarkably well, often with very little scarring on the outside skin probably because the tissues around the vaginal opening are endowed with a rich blood supply. This is convivial to good healing.

A word on birth trauma

Occasionally, tears are pretty extensive and a challenge to repair. If there has been significant trauma caused by childbirth, then the length of time spent recovering may be longer. Luckily, even extensive tears have good prospects of excellent healing without lingering long-term symptoms.

However, I will make mention here that a small number of women with significant tears will end up with an ongoing feeling that their perineum (or pelvic region) is not as strong as before. They have sustained what is being increasingly recognised as birth trauma, where childbirth has resulted in permanent injury of the pelvic floor. Such severe trauma is uncommon but can prove distressing for those affected.

Birth trauma with permanent symptoms happens in a few per cent of all vaginal and instrumental births. It is more likely after a forceps or vacuum birth.

The most common symptoms are bladder weakness (small leaks with sneezing and even vigorous exercise) and vaginal prolapse where the vaginal walls bulge inwards and down towards the vaginal opening. Sometimes there are ongoing bowel symptoms where women feel they have a less secure bowel and flatal control (complete loss of bowel control is very unlikely). The severity of symptoms caused by birth trauma varies greatly.

Birth trauma with ongoing symptoms can involve a fair amount of damage to the muscle attachment to the bony pelvis itself (if you can bear to return to my analogy, it would be as if the sheet of muscle partially detaches from the stadium seating itself, rather than the muscle attachment on the edges of the grassy field which is closer to the vaginal opening). This is a problem because the region where the pelvic floor muscle attaches to the pelvic bone is too deep within the pelvis – too buried under layers of tissues – for us to surgically reattach.

To correct prolapse and bladder continence symptoms gynaecologists have, in the past, reinforced the integrity of the pelvic floor by surgically inserting synthetic mesh. Unfortunately, vaginal mesh (which did produce pretty dramatic improvements in symptoms for some women) has fallen out of favour because it can result in nasty complications. There are still other (non-mesh) surgical options to strengthen the tissues of the perineum, to fix prolapses and improve bladder symptoms. These are variably successful.

The only way to eliminate the risk of birth trauma altogether is to opt for an elective caesar as the planned mode of birth. This is obviously a rather extreme decision if this was the mum-to-be's only concern as the chance of serious birth trauma happening in the first place is low, though we can't predict who it will happen to (I discuss the pros and cons of a planned caesar in Chapter 8).

So, episiotomies and tears are common (and can be easily mended with excellent results), but major birth trauma with permanent problems is *not.* Most tears arising from childbirth will heal fully within weeks without ongoing urinary or bowel symptoms.

Bleeding after birth can sometimes be serious

I introduced you to the concept of micromorts a while back, an unconventional unit of measurement where one micromort equates to one in a million risk of dying.

Just to get your bearings, recall 30 kilometres of walking incurs a risk of 1 micromort (perhaps a freaky scarf-stuck-in-escalator mishap or something else stupidly unlucky for the one in a million who no longer find themselves alive by the end of a leisurely evening stroll). Living two days in New York (air pollution risk), living two months with a smoker (cancer and heart disease risk) or eating 1000 bananas (radioactive potassium-40 risk) all score a 1 micromort risk. A kangaroo encounter scores a 0.1 micromort risk (I suppose it'd be terminal injuries caused by a 1 in 10 million surprise kick from Skippy).

Using this sophisticated mathematical tool, we established that trying to be born is a risky pastime and therefore best chanced once. Although nowhere as dangerous, giving birth is also a somewhat risky venture: childbirth incurs a 170 micromort risk for the mum.

This surprising level of risk is sadly borne out in grim worldwide statistics. World Health Organisation estimated that in 2017, around 295,000 women across the globe did not survive childbirth. Simply harrowing. Most deaths were clustered in low-resource settings, an unspeakable tragedy given most were preventable. Women in the developed world are also at risk, although the absolute risk is small. In the UK in 2017 for instance, there were 7 maternal deaths per 100,000 live births. That's 70 micromorts – the same risk of death as scoffing 70,000 bananas. The risk of death during childbirth is just over three times higher for those in the US compared to the UK, though the overall risk remains very low.

The leading cause of maternal death is catastrophic bleeding after birth – a postpartum haemorrhage.

But do not be anxious. The message I wish to convey is that birth has a bleeding risk that could be life-threatening but, thanks to a host of miraculous lifesaving drugs at our disposal, we can stem the flow before catastrophe strikes. Childbirth in the modern era is very safe.

Why is there bleeding after childbirth?

To nourish a baby of some 3 or so kilograms by the end of pregnancy, mum needs to supply a lot of oxygen and nutrients. To deliver these goodies a lot of mum's blood volume is flowing near the surface of the placenta so bub can be constantly fed. At any one time, 20 per cent of a pregnant person's total blood volume is sloshing about within the uterus.

During pregnancy, the placenta is a physical plug preventing this blood from gushing out from the uterus like a crack in a dam. But when the placenta separates after birth it leaves a large, disc-shaped raw surface on the inner lining of the womb the size of a small pizza. It's from this area that mum can bleed out, with the blood trickling out from the vaginal opening. On occasion it can gush alarmingly briskly.

Nature has built in a system to halt the bleeding. After birth and placental separation there is an almighty uterine contraction, where the womb squeezes into a hard ball. And remains contracted. By doing this, the maternal blood vessels laced throughout the uterine musculature are squished shut. The flow of blood to the exposed surface on the inner lining of the uterus (where the placenta lifted off) stops and the bleeding ceases.

Problems arise if the uterus does not contract down tightly and remains floppy like a deflated balloon – what we call uterine atony. If this happens brisk bleeding continues.

The other major source of bleeding after childbirth is from tears around the vaginal opening, or from episiotomies. This bleeding is arrested by repairing them: the stitching brings the tissues together, putting direct pressure on the edges of the open wound which stops the blood flowing.

Happily, for the majority of pregnancies the combo of the oxytocin injection given just after birth, removing the placenta and stitching tears is all that's needed to stop bleeding before it becomes excessive.

Postpartum haemorrhage

Losses estimated to be less than half a litre is actually considered acceptable blood loss after birth. This is more blood than most are accustomed to seeing (imagine half of a 1 litre milk carton sloshing with blood instead of milk. Not an appetising thing unless your name is Bella or Edward, and you are pale in complexion).

Losses mounting north of 500 millilitres is deemed excessive. Roughly occurring in 5–15 per cent of pregnancies, this situation is called a postpartum haemorrhage and demands urgent action from us.

If the pace of bleeding is concerningly brisk we may call a code, just like what we did when we encountered a different emergency in the prior chapter – a shoulder dystocia. Clinicians will pour into the room to lend assistance – more midwives, obstetricians and perhaps an anaesthetist.

The sudden flurry of frenetic movement may be rather alarming. If it happens in the birth you are involved in, trust the team providing care. Turn your focus to the baby (whether you are the mum or a support person) and do your best not to fret. Also, we understand you may be concerned, but give the clinical staff some time and space to do their thing. Be reassured that in the majority of cases the bleeding is rapidly stemmed within 10 or so minutes, whereupon the emergency code is stood down and the extra helpers shuffle back out of the room.

In most cases it will be a short-lived burst of drama that ends as abruptly as it began.

Steps taken to stop the postpartum bleeding

When there is a postpartum haemorrhage the trained staff is spurred into action. We do two things simultaneously: administer drugs to arrest the bleeding and watch over mum's circulatory system to keep her safe.

We have a slew of drugs we can unleash to stop excessive postpartum bleeding. First, we administer more agents that cajole the uterus to firmly contract, such as a heftier dose of oxytocin which is administered through a drip; or prostaglandin tablets (called misoprostol) inserted into the bottom where it is rapidly absorbed into the bloodstream.

A very important drug we can deploy is ergometrine. Like oxytocin, it is injected into the thigh or via the drip. But unlike oxytocin which acts on uterine muscles, ergometrine acts directly on the walls of blood vessels and clamps them shut.

It is fascinating to note that historical accounts reveal 'ergot' was used by (evidently very cluey) midwives for centuries. In 1935, two chemists – C Moir and H Dudley – purified ergot and developed the drug ergometrine. It has been argued that this humble drug – cheap, accessible yet still unheard of by many – is an unsung hero that has saved a staggering number of lives. Its use is perhaps a major reason why there has been an impressive fall in maternal deaths from childbirth across the 20th century (you may note that it was developed during the same decade when gulping down castor oil was in vogue as a futile way to kickstart labour).

Oddly, ergometrine is also an essential ingredient for LSD. It boggles my brain how anyone would even guess that a drug used to stem bleeding during childbirth could be remotely useful as an ingredient to produce a recreational drug with hallucinogenic properties; one that can assist youngsters to manically dance all night at rave parties (and can be sold in dimly lit alleyways for tidy sums).

We may also give another remarkable drug called tranexamic acid. This drug works by encouraging blood to clot, which slows the flow; similar in concept to the fact that mangey tuffs of hair caught in the strainer slows water escaping from a shower. We give it as an intravenous injection to treat postpartum haemorrhage, but some may be familiar with tranexamic acid as a tablet taken to alleviate heavy periods.

Tranexamic acid was discovered in the 1950s by an inspirational Japanese female academic by the name of Utako Okamoto. Professor Okamoto obsessed in finding a drug to counter bleeding after childbirth. What was terribly tragic – for her and for the many lives the drug could have saved – is that for decades tranexamic acid was prevented from seeing the light of day by the overwhelmingly male-dominated academic environment of her era. In an interview recorded in 2012, she recounted that she was once asked to leave a medical conference because the event was not for 'women and children'. In another shameful incident, after presenting her discovery Okamoto was asked by male audience members whether she was going to dance for them. Consequently, the lifesaving potential of tranexamic acid remained cloaked from view for years and it was only in 2010 – some five decades after its discovery – that an enormous clinical trial testing the drug (called the WOMAN trial) was commenced. Recruiting some 20,000 women at 200 hospitals across 21 countries, the trial confirmed tranexamic acid saves women dying from heavy bleeding at childbirth. Professor Okamoto knew about this clinical trial commencing, but she sadly died at the age of 98 before hearing of the positive findings.

Although Okamoto originally developed the drug for postpartum bleeding, another clinical trial showed her amazing invention also saves people exsanguinating from major trauma. Put simply, Professor Okamoto is a hero.

Thus, with the onset of a bleed we may administer tranexamic acid, ergometrine and oxytocin through a drip; and prostaglandin tablets into the rectum (or inject a powerful prostaglandin through the drip). In quick succession. These drugs will be enough to turn off the tap for the large majority of bleeds.

Besides giving drugs, a midwife or doctor will place a hand on mum's tummy to massage the uterus. This direct stimulation on the uterus encourages it to contract, which can also help stop the bleeding.

Watching mum's circulatory system to keep her safe

Even though we are taking all these measures to stop the bleeding, we need to keep mum safe.

As you might imagine, losing too much fluid from the circulatory system is unsafe. We don't wait to let this happen, of course. To protect mum, we put in a drip so we can directly access her circulatory system. We then watch her like a hawk and replace fluid losses as required.

Mum's circulation will have no problems tolerating the typical losses that arise from most cases of postpartum bleeding. Pregnant women start with a total circulatory volume of about 6–7 litres, meaning their bodies can comfortably cope with losses of around a litre. Even so, we don't like losses to stray much beyond this or her circulatory system may start becoming unstable. A blood pressure that suddenly drops, or a pulse that starts to race, are clues that her body is starting to seriously strain from excessive blood loss.

To keep the circulation filled we run sterile salty water through the drip. Often this is all that's needed to stabilise mum's circulatory system and to keep her safe. For really serious bleeding we may give donated blood products through the drip. We give blood very sparingly and only a minority of postpartum bleeds will need it. But when there is very severe bleeding, replacing blood with blood can be lifesaving.

The next steps if bleeding persists

For a very small proportion of cases, blood continues to trickle despite all these steps. When the estimated blood loss is well over a litre and there are no signs that the bleeding is abating, we will move mum to the operating theatre to try other things.

The anaesthetist will put mum to sleep. Then we first do what is called an 'examination under anaesthesia'. We place a gloved hand inside the womb and feel along the walls to make sure there are no remnants of placenta still clinging on. Small chunks left behind can tent open the inner cavity of the womb which causes persistent bleeding.

Being in theatre is an opportunity for us to do a careful inspection of the vaginal walls higher up. A pesky tear deep within the vagina can also be a reason for recalcitrant bleeding and a few well-placed stitches can sort this out (high vaginal tears can be too difficult to mend in the birth suite as the lighting and equipment is nowhere as good as in the operating theatre).

If there is still bleeding we can insert a specialised balloon inside the cavity of the womb, one that's much larger than that used to ripen the cervix (one we often use is called a 'Bakri balloon'). Once filled, the balloon pushes against the inner walls of the uterus, providing direct pressure to stop the bleeding. Just like how we apply pressure on a bleeding pimple with a tissue (which we might have 'accidentally' picked the top off, only to unleash a miniaturised volcano of blood).

Rarely, these measures still do not stop the bleeding. Our next step is to make a surgical incision on the abdomen (like a caesar) to directly access the uterus. We are then only left with two options.

We can put in a 'B-Lynch suture', which is a technique where we place stitches that wrap around the uterus and squish it down tightly. It's a little like braces worn on formal men's clothing and it is hoped that the physical squeeze of the uterus will arrest the flow.

If all these measures fail, the bleeding dribbles on, and on – estimated losses have strayed into the many litres – and we are getting very worried about the safety of the mum, then the only choice left is a hysterectomy. We do not make such a decision lightly. It is the last resort option to save a life. Crummy when it happens. Luckily, the extreme step of a hysterectomy to stop massive postpartum bleeding is hardly ever done – only once in every few thousand births.

A final word on postpartum bleeding

I realise this book has taken a dark, serious turn. I am sorry about this.

Here I wish to reassure you by providing perspective. Yes, postpartum bleeding does happen, but the vast majority of cases settle quickly, most within minutes. A visit to theatre is most uncommon and losing the womb to postpartum bleeding is just darn rare.

Please trust the clinical team providing care if postpartum bleeding arises. You may see us darting about quickly and the birthing room may be suddenly buzzing with staff. But don't mistake speed for chaos and panic. We know what we are doing and have expertly dealt with this situation many times before. Let the skilled team of midwives and doctors do what they need to do so they can get on top of the bleeding quickly. To keep mum safe.

If we succeeded with plan A – vaginal birth – our trip is at an end. Congratulations all round.

We have now arrived at a truly special moment. The clinical staff have vacated the room, leaving mum, newborn (swaddled or naked) in her arms, spouse (or birth partner) and perhaps a few others dear to mum.

The room is now quiet. Just gentle cooing from a baby becoming familiar with its own voice.

During this brief snapshot in time this newborn is secret, known only to the privileged few in the room (the staff are sworn to secrecy and aren't blabbing to anyone). It is a golden moment to savour. A fleeting window where pure innocence is untouched by social media.

When you arrive at this moment, I'd like to make an earnest suggestion: resist the impulse to immediately announce the birth to the world. Just for a bit. Take photos, but don't text. Cuddle the baby, but don't phone. Chat amongst yourselves, but don't make it 'Facebook official'. Just not yet.

Instead, take a few moments to breathe in this truly rare occasion with full attention – for you are living the memory you will embrace lifelong. Make it last.

Let those beyond the walls of the room wait a little longer for the happy tidings. Text one person and in an instant, the virtual world will be set ablaze. Within a blink, everyone in the room will be jolted back into the zombie world of screens, thumbing their phones to read well wishes from the afar. Everyone except the baby. And the unique moment will be lost forever.

I am afraid we aren't quite done with exploring the possible roads to childbirth. We don't always arrive at a vaginal birth. The last century has witnessed a dramatic fall in the death of babies during labour because of two lifesaving interventions: caesarean sections and instrumental births. Over the next two chapters, I cover why they're done and how they're done safely.

Recap:
The third stage of labour

1. The third stage is defined as the time between birth of the baby and delivery of the placenta. In most cases, the placenta slides out within 15 minutes after the baby. Though occasionally, it can take up to an hour.

2. For around 2–3 per cent of births, the placenta cannot be coaxed to let go of the uterus. What's called a 'retained placenta'. When this happens, we may need to take mum for a brief visit to the operating theatre and perform a manual removal of placenta. We don a long glove, reach in and take out the placenta from the uterus. It's a hassle, but it's safe and quick.

3. If there are vaginal tears, or we performed an episiotomy, we will mend them straight after the birth using stitches that will dissolve on their own. Please be reassured that most tears will heal promptly with excellent results. In general, the region around the vaginal opening heals remarkably well with very minimal scarring.

4. Sometimes tears injure the anal sphincter, the ring of muscle that allows us to control our bowels. If this is the case, it will need careful repair and we often choose to do this in the operating theatre because it is better set up to perform specialised procedures.

5. In a few per cent of vaginal births, tearing can be pretty extensive where recovery can take awhile. And for a small number of women whose pelvic floor muscles have been significantly injured during childbirth, there may be a degree of permanent pelvic floor weakness.

6. Up to 500 millilitres of bleeding is considered normal. Losses that are higher than this is considered excessive, what's called postpartum bleeding. If it happens we will take steps to stem the flow by giving drugs to make the uterus squeeze tightly, or a drug that encourages blood to clot. Also, we will put in an intravenous drip and we may run fluids through it to keep mum safe. On occasion, we may offer donated blood through the drip to replace losses.

7. For a very small number of women with postpartum bleeding these drugs are unable to stop the trickle. When the blood loss is estimated to be well over a litre and the bleeding refuses to abate, we may move mum to the operating theatre to try some different things to stop the flow. If none of these measures stop the bleeding the only final recourse is a hysterectomy. But be reassured this drastic step is only taken for one in every few thousand births. It's really rare.

8. Please bear in mind that most of the things listed here do not happen (other than small tears that require mending, that's pretty common). Be reassured that in most cases, the placenta slides out without controversy, bleeding is minimal, we may or (or may not) put in a few stitches...and childbirth is well and truly over.

Chapter 7

A helping hand: birth by forceps or the vacuum

If the second stage is reached, assisting birth either by forceps or vacuum (or a ventouse) becomes an option whenever there is a compelling reason to expedite birth. Around one in four first-time mums in Australia will have an instrumental birth. It's about the same rate in the UK but is considerably less in the US. The good news is that for those who have birthed vaginally before (even if by forceps or ventouse) the chances of a normal vaginal birth next time lift sharply.

Given instrumental births are fairly common, here we will explore this path to childbirth.

A triple obstetrical tragedy

It's a quirky fact that an ill-fated decision, once upon a time, to not use the obstetric forceps gave the world Prince Charles. And by association, Camilla Parker Bowles. And all the entertaining shenanigans of Prince Harry.

On 3 November 1817, Princess Charlotte of Wales broke her waters and started labouring. Her obstetrician, Sir Richard Croft, no doubt felt a burdensome weight of responsibility. Not only because he was tasked with caring for two royal lives but also of keeping afloat the hopes of all England, the world's most dominant nation (commanding a quarter of the world's population). Aged only 21, Princess Charlotte of Wales was the daughter of the future King George the IV, destined to inherit the throne and adored by her subjects.

Over the tense months leading to 3 November, Sir Richard probably spent a fair bit of time praying (day and night) that Princess Charlotte's destiny was to be a speedy birth, just like Alice in vignette one – our lucky friend from the Introduction. He may have even dared ponder the lavish rewards that might be bestowed upon him by a grateful Monarch. A prime parcel of land perhaps? Not a third rate, sludgy marshland but a lush estate with miles of green hills undulating into the picturesque horizon, dotted with deer bounding about under perfect sunsets.

I am afraid a straightforward vaginal birth for the princess wasn't on the cards. Not even close. For starters, the first stage of labour dribbled on for a harrowing 26 hours (with no effective painkillers on offer, not even a sterile water injection).

Then things really went pear shaped. The second stage lasted for 24 hours, which is just not a thing in modern obstetrics. During all this time Sir Richard decided against using the forceps. A relatively new tool, it was not in favour among the British medical establishment. He must have really angst over this decision because he was skilled in its use. In fact, he was taught the art of the forceps by the highly regarded London obstetrician Thomas Denman. Denman had a 'law' that the forceps be applied after the head had rested for six hours on the perineum.

Tragically, after being trapped in the second stage of labour for literally a day, Princess Charlotte passed a stillborn infant. Horrifically, death soon followed for the princess herself. Probably owing to the unspeakably long labour, she died five hours after her newborn – exsanguinating from massive postpartum bleeding. The date of her death was recorded as 6 November 1817, days after labour had begun. A brutal way to succumb for a young woman in her early twenties who had a long regal life to look forward to.

Charlotte's death triggered immense grief among the British, who had held her as a golden ray of hope to save them from her deeply unpopular grandfather (King George III) and her equally loathed father (future king George IV). She was the only legitimate grandchild of the current king. As a result, this obstetric tragedy tipped off a major rejig in the line of royal succession. Sensing opportunity, the King's unmarried sons stirred into action and competed to produce a successor to the throne. Eventually, the fourth son (Prince Edward, Duke of Kent and Strathearn) fathered the future heir to the monarchy, the majestic Queen Victoria – the very sovereign who inhaled chloroform to ease the pain of childbirth back in Chapter 2, and Prince Charles's great-great-great-grandmother (and, I suppose, Carmilla Parker Bowles' great-great-great-grandmother in-law).

What may have further wounded poor Sir Richard Croft is that Thomas Denman – the obstetric authority who taught him how to use the forceps – was also his father-in-law. Perhaps mercifully, Denman died two years before this incident, which no doubt spared Sir Richard from cruel in-law jibes. ('Six hours, then apply forceps. I told you! If only they had asked *me* to care for the princess…')

Improbably, the tale gets worse. Sir Richard's spirits never recovered from this workplace misadventure. He spiralled into despair. His patients deserted him. He remained unconsoled by an enquiry conducted by two other sirs who cleared his good name (there were evidently a lot of knights back then). They concluded that everything had been done 'for the best'.

On 13 February 1818, three months after the auspicious tragedy, Sir Richard was called upon to attend the birth of Mrs Thackeray (wife of Reverend Dr Thackeray) at their residence. It became clear that labour was not progressing well. Sir Richard, possibly lacking self-confidence, became deeply agitated. When members of the family expressed anxiety as to how it was all going, he struck his forehead and shot back, 'What is your agitation compared to mine?' (This sort of behaviour does not generally inspire confidence in patients – the poor chap had clearly lost it).

At midnight he retired to a guest room one floor above that where Mrs Thackeray continued to labour. It was also where Dr Thackeray kept two pistols in a drawer. At around 1 o'clock in the morning the Thackerays' servant heard a noise. She went to check in on Sir Richard, rapped on his door and took a glance. What she saw is dramatically encapsulated in this original quote from an 1818 newspaper piece: 'The body of Sir Richard Croft was lying on the bed shockingly mangled…both (pistols) were discharged, and the head of the unfortunate gentleman was literally blown to pieces.'

When the coroner visited the scene, he noticed a copy of Shakespeare's Love's Labour's Lost perched on the chair by the bedstead. It was opened on the following passage (Act V, Scene II): 'Fair Sir, God Save you! Where is the Princess?'

And just to spell out what a ludicrously cursed soul Sir Richard was, had he held his nerve he would have witnessed a happy outcome. Around eight in the morning, Mrs Thackeray was safely delivered by Mr Herbert, Sir Croft's occasional assistant.

This horrid tale of Sir Croft has been dubbed 'The triple obstetrical tragedy': the loss of mother, baby and doctor.

It's thought that the forceps popped into existence some 300–400 years ago. Forceps (and subsequently caesars) replaced a terrible procedure called a craniotomy, done when it was clear that baby was never coming out vaginally (presumably after an unspeakably long second stage). Performed to save the mother and practised since the mists of time across many cultures, a craniotomy is a destructive procedure and let's leave it at that.

Whether or not it's true, credit for the discovery of the forceps falls to one dynastic family – a rather eccentric one by the name of Chamberlen. They were peculiar in at least two respects. First, they had a singular lack of imagination when choosing names for their offspring. The first Chamberlen, William (d 1959), was a surgeon in Paris who moved rather quickly to London to flee from religious persecution (a rather common pastime throughout European history). William imaginatively named his sons Peter the Elder and Peter the Younger. Peter the Younger then named his son Peter. Peter – by this, I mean Peter the Younger's son and nephew of Peter the Elder – then had a son Hugh Senior. Hugh Senior then had a son, Hugh Junior.

The second odd thing about the Chamberlens is that having discovered a ground-breaking invention that could save a lot of lives, all these Peters and Hughs decided they ought to keep the forceps a closely guarded family secret. For over a century.

We believe this was possible because modesty dictated that whenever a male accoucheur attended a birth, he would do so under a drape. This means he, and any secretive tools he may have spirited under this snug tent, would remain hidden from view.

Just like the identities of the herbs and spices that transforms KFC chicken into such mouth-watering lingual pleasures, some secrets are too good to forever conceal. The forceps were eventually outed and are now widely available.

The reasons why instrumental births are done

The villains responsible for caesars during the first stage of labour – fetal distress and arrested labour (or 'failure to progress') – are the main reasons why we resort to instrumental births during the second stage. You can flick back to read more about this in Chapter 5.

Active pushing adds further stress to the baby on top of the strain caused by uterine contractions. Hence, during pushing it is quite common to see fetal heart rate patterns acutely worsen because the fetus isn't getting the oxygen it needs. Happily, with robust pushing there is often steady progression of the baby down the birth canal that leads to a vaginal birth. But not always. For labours where the second stage is protracted – not uncommon for first-time mums – the use of forceps or the vacuum to expedite birth can occasionally be lifesaving. If we stubbornly wait for a vaginal birth, this can significantly increase the length of time that babies are left languishing in a suffocating environment. As a result, some will arrive in very poor condition and require heavy-duty resuscitation efforts. And a fraction of them will not do well at all.

Arrested labour, or 'failure to progress', is apparent if the baby has not arrived after a long period of pushing. It's far more likely to happen to first-time mums and is uncommon for experienced mums who have birthed vaginally before (even if their prior birth was assisted by forceps, or ventouse).

The duration we can safely ask women to continue actively pushing before making the call of arrested labour, and proceeding with an instrumental birth, is surprisingly unresolved. Most countries wait until women have actively pushed around one to two hours before recommending an instrumental birth, and I think that's about right. Interestingly, in the United States it is widespread practice to encourage women to actively push for three or so hours before an instrumental birth is offered.

The obvious benefit if we encourage women to push a very, very long time (as they do in the States) is that they may, of course, have a better chance of having a vaginal birth and avoiding an instrumental birth altogether. Indeed, forceps and ventouses are used considerably less often in the US compared to Australia, United Kingdom and many parts of Europe. This is good.

However, there are important drawbacks for women left pushing for hours upon hours. Firstly, a prolonged period of active pushing lengthens the time that baby is left in a stressful uterine environment. This increases the likelihood that the baby comes out flat, requiring sturdy resuscitation efforts.

Secondly, if pushing has dribbled on for ages but the baby fails to emerge and a caesar is required (yes, caesars can still happen during the second stage, as we will find out soon), the protracted period of pushing will have rendered the uterine tissues fragile. Although a caesar can still be safely done, a really long labour makes the operation more hazardous with a higher chance of significant blood loss.

A very long period spent in the second stage also increases the risk of significant postpartum bleeding after the birth. This is probably because the uterine muscle is simply exhausted after epically long labours and is too tired to contract tightly into a ball during the third stage.

Finally, over the entire period of full cervical dilatation the baby's head is deep within the pelvis and gives the muscles of the pelvic floor a terrific stretch. An exceptionally long time spent in the second stage may have lasting impacts on mum's pelvic floor. Indeed, large epidemiological studies have made a link between the length of time spent in the second stage of labour and the chances of developing vaginal wall prolapse and bladder complaints in later life.

Most countries abide by a rule of permitting active pushing to go for one to two hours before offering an instrumental birth. Others encourage women to push for a third hour. I suggest you go with whatever your birth suite does as they will have finely honed their clinical skills with an approach that they are most familiar with (and if you are in The States, I hope you have had your Wheaties).

How forceps births are done

It will be comforting that the same doctor and midwife providing care during the first stage (whom you have gotten to know and trust) will often be the ones facilitating the forceps birth. Others may also be in the room, such as other midwives or doctors on tap to lend a hand. We may invite a paediatric doctor to discreetly stand in the corner, just in case the newborn needs resuscitation.

We place mum into the lithotomy position: on her back in bed (with her body semi-upright at a 45-degree angle), legs raised in the air by padded holders under her calves, and her thighs rotated out. The obstetrician performing the forceps will be standing (or sitting) in front of the vaginal opening.

The forceps are shaped like salad servers that snuggly wrap around the baby's head. It's made up of two 'blades' almost identical in shape (there is a left and right, just like shoes). When slid in place a blade neatly sits on either side of the baby's head, grasping it firmly (imagine salad servers grasping a lemon, which represents the head). Once in position each blade runs down from on top of the head, curves along the side of the head around the ears and ends by hugging the baby's cheeks. The other end that continues beyond the top of the baby's head comes together as a thin shaft that emerges out the vagina and terminate as handles that the obstetrician can grasp. Once the blades are gently placed around the baby's head they lock together at the shaft and become one instrument.

We will first numb the tissues of the vaginal opening by performing what's called a pudendal block. We inject local anaesthetic in a specific spot about 5 centimetres within the vagina (near bony landmarks that are part of mum's pelvic bone called the 'ischial spines', which you will hear more about soon). The injection blocks a nerve – the pudendal nerve – that supplies pain fibres around the vaginal opening. We may also inject local anaesthetic directly into the skin at the vaginal opening just in case we perform an episiotomy. If there is an epidural on board these injections aren't needed.

The obstetrician will slide the blades of the forceps around the baby's head one by one – eased in with a light touch. While this is happening, you may catch a glimpse of the metal blades of the forceps and be alarmed by their size. And perhaps intimidated by their metallic-ness. But try not to be. They are actually quite thin when viewed side on. They just need to be the length they are for reach.

For a forceps birth we usually time the pull of the forceps with mum's pushing efforts. Mum still needs to push just as hard as before. And once we start using the forceps the baby is birthed within two or three sets of contractions: it is not safe for us to keep tugging away if the baby hasn't appeared by this time. While the baby's head is crowning, we may perform an episiotomy.

The important thing to know (and be reassured about) is that we do not pull the forceps with brute force. That is not good technique. Some force is applied for sure, but the forceps' role is mainly to guide the baby's head around the final curve of the pelvis and lift it into the outside world. If the head is very close to the vaginal opening the obstetrician will not be pulling with much force at all. Mum pushes, and we steer.

Once the head is out, we slip the forceps off and deliver the rest of the baby just like a vaginal birth. We can also plonk junior straight on mum's tummy. However, if a forceps births was performed because we were concerned about the condition of the baby (we were prompted by worrying fetal heart rate patterns seen on the CTG) we may pass the baby straight to the paediatric doctor for a check in the resuscitation area. If all is well – baby is breathing, pink and perhaps crying – then bubby will be promptly returned to mum for hugs, kisses and cuddles.

Vacuum (ventouse) births

The vacuum – also known as the ventouse – is very similar in concept to forceps in that it's another way to grab hold of the baby so it can be pulled out to expedite birth. But instead of something that wraps around bub's head, the ventouse is a suction cup placed on the head. Rather like a vacuum cleaner sucking on a bowling ball (aka the baby's head).

The suction cup of the ventouse is a shallow disc some 5–7 centimetres across and 3 centimetres in thickness. We slide the cup on the head (the back of the head in fact, not right on the top, as this encourages the head to remain nicely flexed where the face is tucked into the chest). Emerging from the centre of the cup is a long, thin, flexible cord that runs out of the vaginal opening to a handle held by the obstetrician.

The handle has a pump and once the cup is in place, we manually pump up the suction. This generates a strong negative pressure within the suction cup (500–600 mmHg for the physics-minded). The section of junior's scalp beneath the cup is sucked in and fills the space within the cup, creating what's called a 'chignon'. I note this because when babies have just birthed assisted by the ventouse, they will have a raised, disc-shaped section on their scalp. This little 'hat' is expected, not dangerous and disappears within a day or so.

Once the cup is in place and the suction is on, we perform a ventouse-assisted birth similarly to a forceps birth. We time our pulls with uterine contractions and maternal pushing. Again, we aim for birth to happen within three sets of contractions. And once the head is out, we switch off the suction (by pressing a button on the handle), remove the ventouse then deliver the rest of the baby.

You may be wondering how we choose between the forceps or the ventouse? For the most part it depends on the clinician; some are simply trained to use one over the other. Oddly, it also depends on which country the mum is giving birth. Both the ventouse and forceps are used in Australia and the UK, whereas Israel and Sweden do not use forceps at all.

I do suggest you let the clinician use whichever they are most comfortable with and most skilled at.

Critical information we gather before an instrumental birth – how low is the head, and which way is bubby facing?

The obstetrician starts by performing a vaginal examination to determine the type of instrumental birth to do, and the likely level of difficulty. This is a critical assessment – wielded incorrectly, forceps or the ventouse can be dangerous.

The doctor is gathering two vital pieces of information: how far the head has descended down the birth canal (the lower, the safer) and the direction the baby is facing (occipital anterior position is the easiest). Let's explore each in turn.

How low is the head? Mid-cavity vs a low instrumental birth

Instrumental births are straightforward if the head is low down in the birth canal, but far more challenging if it is still high.

To figure out how low the head is, we feel where the lowermost edge of baby's bony skull sits in relation to fixed bony points on mum's bony pelvis – subtle protuberances called the 'ischial spines'. These spines are felt through the vaginal skin. There is one on either side and they lurk 5 centimetres from the vaginal opening. Being bony and unyielding, they represent a reliable fixed point along the birth canal to judge how far the baby's head is from the outside world.

If the baby's head has descended to the level of 'the spines' but is no lower, it's still 5 centimetres from the vaginal opening. That's too high to safely attempt an instrumental birth. If an urgent delivery is called for, a caesar is the safest option even though the cervix is fully dilated. Attempting a 'high forceps' to wrench out a baby when the head is so high is dangerous because it is uncertain whether it will fit through the pelvis. In fact, if the head remains so high after a long period of active pushing it should raise suspicions that mum's pelvis may be too narrow for the baby. If so, jamming on the forceps and tugging hard could cause nasty injuries.

In contrast, if the head is really low – say 3 centimetres below the spines (meaning 2 centimetres shy of the vaginal opening) or beyond – we deem this a 'low instrumental' birth. These are very safe and only require the gentlest of pulls by the obstetrician or doctor performing the procedure. Luckily, in most cases where a forceps or ventouse is called for, the head will be low enough for a 'low instrumental birth'.

If the head has descended to be between 0 and 2 centimetres below the ischial spines, it sits in a grey zone of the 'mid-cavity'. The choices are to perform a caesar at full dilatation or attempt what is called a mid-cavity instrumental birth. Mid-cavity instrumental births are challenging. They are best performed – or supervised – by an experienced obstetrician.

When we undertake a mid-cavity instrumental birth there is a chance the forceps or ventouse does not succeed in delivering the baby vaginally. If we start the instrumental birth and decide it is safest to stop trying, we will convert to a caesarean section immediately.

Switching over to a caesar after a few attempts at a mid-cavity instrumental birth certainly does not mean there has been a failure of good clinical judgement or that the obstetrician isn't good. In fact, it is a critical skill of experienced obstetricians to judge whether it is safe to continue attempting the mid-cavity instrumental birth or to abandon further attempts (knowing to stop). We figure this out by feeling whether there is any head descent during the pulls. If we sense there is absolutely no movement with a decent pull (as though the other end of the forceps is concreted in a brick wall), we will stop attempting the instrumental birth and convert to a caesarean section. Obstetricians should not try to overcome the lack of descent by pulling harder; this is a pitfall for inexperienced doctors (that will not be your doctor, of course). Some babies stuck in the mid-cavity may just be too big to safely pass through the pelvis where a forceful yank could result in significant injuries to the baby or the mother.

Because of the risk of converting to a caesar, we often move mum to the operating theatre before attempting a mid-cavity instrumental birth. This allows us to rapidly switch over to a caesar if needed because once we start pulling on the baby's head, it becomes time critical to get baby out. This is because the tugs themselves add considerable stress to the baby (another reason why overcoming a lack of descent by pulling much harder is a terrible idea). Promptly converting to a caesar is not an immediate option if an unsuccessful instrumental attempt has been made in the birth suite, distant from the operating theatre.

I've said a lot here about mid-cavity instrumental births, but most will be low instrumental births, which are straightforward. The ventouse or forceps are put on the baby's head in the birth suite and we gently pull while mum gives a few final pushes. Very quickly the baby emerges, nice and healthy.

Which way is the baby facing? Rotational instrumental birth

The other thing the obstetrician assesses by vaginal examination before embarking on an instrumental birth is the way baby is facing. The easiest (and safest) instrumental birth by far is when the baby's head is not only low but in the occipital anterior position. If you don't mind me harking back to our marine analogy, occipital anterior is where our (by now, seriously bewildered) fish is swimming through the birth canal the 'right way up' – eyeballs closer to mum's pubic bone, mouth closer to mum's anus (baby facing towards mum's back).

The degree of difficulty for the instrumental birth increases considerably if baby is in the occipital transverse (facing sideways, the baby eyeballs closer to one thigh and the mouth closer to the opposite thigh) or occipital posterior (where the baby is upside down – eyeballs closer to mum's anus and its mouth towards the sky, just under the pubic bone).

Delivering babies in the occipital transverse (sideways facing) or occipital posterior (upside down) positions requires a rotational instrumental birth. Like mid-cavity instrumental births, they are harder to do and calls for a higher level of obstetric skill.

The aim of a rotational instrumental birth is to swivel the head to the correct occipital anterior position. It's a 90-degree turn for babies starting in the occipital transverse position and 180 degrees for those in the occipital posterior position. Once the head has rotated to the occipital anterior position the baby is then pulled down through the birth canal and is birthed.

The reason we need to turn the baby to the occipital anterior position is that this is the orientation where the baby presents the smallest diameter to squeeze through the final length of the birth canal. When in the occipital anterior position, the baby will naturally flex neck the most effectively so that its chin is tucked deeply onto its chest. In contrast, when in the occipital transverse (aka sideways fish) or occipital posterior position (aka upside-down fish) the head does not fit snugly through.

There are a few options to rotate the baby. We can apply the ventouse (called a rotational ventouse); we can use a gloved hand to swivel the head to the occipital anterior position (called a manual rotation) then apply the forceps to pull the baby out; or we can use Kielland's forceps which are specifically designed to rotate babies to the occipital anterior orientation (the Kielland's are applied and twirled around so the head is spun to the occipital anterior position before being birthed). The obstetrician will select the technique they are trained to do and are most comfortable with.

Similar to a mid-cavity forceps, we may sometimes attempt the rotational instrumental birth in the operating theatre because there is a chance we are unable to birth the baby through the vagina (this then allows us to rapidly deliver the baby by caesar). But not always: rotational instrumental births can be safely done in the birth suite if the head is very low down the birth canal as the likelihood of success is very high.

The risks with instrumental births

Before we touch on the sensitive issue of risk, please bear in mind that the majority of forceps or ventouse births happen without complications.

Uncommonly, birth assisted by forceps or the ventouse can injure the baby. Although distressing if it happens, most injuries are minor and the baby quickly recovers. Less concerning injuries include a type of scalp trauma called a 'cephalohaematoma'. Occurring in around 10 per cent of ventouse births, there is a confined secondary bleed within the scalp, like a big bruise. Most disappear within days. Forceps may cause bruising to the face, but this also promptly disappears.

Very uncommonly, instrumental births can cause more serious injuries. These include a skull fracture (more with forceps than the ventouse); a confined bleed into the brain (most recover, it's not like strokes that adults get); and even seizures (though I would note if a seizure happens after an instrumental birth it can be difficult to deduce whether the forceps were responsible or because very low oxygen levels in the womb caused it, in which case the forceps actually saved the baby from further serious harm).

Please be reassured the likelihood that such serious injuries happen to the baby after an instrumental birth are very low – less than half a per cent. In keeping with the fact that they are harder to do, these risks are higher with mid-cavity or rotational instrumental births but even so, the overall probability remains very low. And even if these serious injuries arise, modern neonatal medicine can nurse nearly all these babies back to perfect health. Permanent injury caused by forceps or the ventouse is rare.

You may recall that vaginal birth incurs a risk of pelvic floor injury, including a tear through the anal sphincter (a third-degree tear). The risk is higher after instrumental births, particularly with mid-cavity and rotational instrumental births. It does happen and isn't altogether rare. And as discussed before, we can fix anal sphincter tears with good outcomes.

Forceps and vacuums have saved untold lives. And prevented many cases of permanent brain injury caused by babies trapped in a suffocating bind of catastrophically low oxygen.

I hope the knowledge you gleaned from this chapter will be helpful should an instrumental birth be fated as part of your future birth experience. You now know why we do them and how they're done; that once we begin them it doesn't take long before baby emerges; and that a majority are done with a light touch and have excellent outcomes.

Friend, we are getting close to the end of our time together. Only one more small thing to cover and you can set down this book and return to regular viewing (a foreign language Netflix series perhaps? The offerings from South Korea can be really zany and fun to watch).

In the next chapter we will explore the escape hatch, the abdominal zipper, the sun roof…the mighty caesarean section.

Recap:
Birth assisted by forceps or the ventouse

1. The main reasons why instrumental births (forceps or ventouse) are done is because of fetal distress (where we are concerned that oxygen levels in the fetus may be worryingly low); or arrested labour ('failure to progress') where the baby has not emerged after a long period of spirited pushing.

2. For instrumental births mum is placed in the lithotomy position – body semi-upright, legs raised in the air by padded holders under her calves, and her thighs rotated out.

3. Forceps is an instrument that snuggly wraps around the baby's head. A ventouse (or vacuum) is a round suction disc applied to the baby's head. The strong suction within the disc produces a round, raised section of scalp at birth that disappears within a day or so. We pull on the forceps, or ventouse, during contractions while mum pushes. Once we start the procedure the baby is usually birthed within three sets of contractions.

4. It is important to know (and be reassured) that we do not pull on the forceps, or ventouse, with brute force. That's not good technique. Some force is applied but the aim is to help guide the head around the final curve of the birth canal and lift it into the outside world.

5. If the head has already descended far down the birth canal and is very close to being born, the instrumental birth will usually be straightforward and entails very little risk ('low instrumental birth'). In such cases the pull is particularly gentle, and we are really only guiding the baby's head.

6. Instrumental births can be rather more challenging if the head is higher up in the birth canal, or the baby is not facing the right way (not in the optimal 'occipital anterior' position – eyes closer to mum's pubic bone, mouth closer to the mum's anus). These may require more experienced obstetricians to attend the birth.

7. Sometimes the obstetrician anticipates the instrumental birth may be challenging and cannot be sure whether they can safely get the baby out through the vagina. In such cases they may decide it's best to attempt the procedure in the operative suite. This is because if they are unable to perform the instrumental birth, they can swiftly proceed to a caesarean section to deliver the bub safely.

8. There are some risks with instrumental births. They can cause minor bruising to the scalp or face, but this will harmlessly disappear within days. Very uncommonly (half a per cent), they can cause more serious injuries that take longer to mend. But be reassured that it's rare for the forceps, or ventouse, to cause permanent injury to the baby.

9. Like vaginal births, pelvic floor injury can be caused by instrumental births. We can mend them, and most have

good outcomes. Uncommonly, the injury can be more serious and needs a longer time to heal.

10. Please bear in mind that instrumental births are largely very safe. Over the centuries they have saved the lives of untold numbers of babies.

Chapter 8

The sunroof exit: birth by caesarean section

The caesar has become a standing item of hot politics and stirred up a tremendous hoo-ha. Many would argue it's the safest way for babies to be born as it bypasses the suffocating stress that can arise from uterine contractions during labour that we've heard all about. At the same time, it is deeply maligned by others as an unnatural cop-out and enthusiastically demonised as a man-made evil to assiduously avoid – an operation abused by trigger happy obstetricians that disempowers women by robbing them of the experience of a vaginal birth. And often done more for the convenience of doctors rather than the sake of babies or mothers. Doctors, hospitals, regions and whole nations are named and slandered for their 'disgracefully' high caesar rates.

The caesarean section is the most common operation in the world. Variations in rates between nations are astounding. In 2015, 26 per cent births in the United Kingdom were by caesar. Although this may seem high, it is only half the rate seen in Egypt, Turkey and Brazil where around 55 per cent of babies are born by caesar. Thirty-three per cent of births in the United States were by caesarean section but only 14 per cent in the Netherlands, and yet bad infant outcomes are similar in both countries.

What is the 'right' number of caesars? There isn't likely to be a single percentage that neatly applies to all countries; 15–20 per cent is probably the lower end that's needed to save a majority of babies from the stress of labour. Rates of caesars in many Pacific Island nations are in low single digits but sadly, the percentage of babies dying as a result of pregnancy are also in low single digits (losses in well-resourced nations are ten-fold less). Once rates of caesars for large populations stray north of 25–30 per cent, further gains in baby survival for every percentage point increase are likely to become smaller and smaller. Many lives would be saved if a nation had the resources to lift its caesarean rate from 5 per cent to 20 per cent, but far less babies would be saved if a well-resourced country with a baseline caesar rate of 30 per cent increased it to 45 per cent (though there would probably still be some additional babies saved). Everyone will draw different lines in the sand, and I do not believe there can be an absolute truth.

Let others debate where the line sits. Let us only worry about the one special birth you will soon be a part of. In this final bit of the book, you will learn all about the caesar, just in case it ends up being part of your birth experience.

Then, my young Padawan, your training is at an end.

Reasons for having a caesar

Caesars done during labour are called emergency caesars and our familiar foes, fetal distress and arrested labour (or 'failure to progress'), are the main reason why they are done. If these evils befall a labour during the first stage then a caesar is the only option to expedite birth. If the second stage is reached then – as we chewed on in the previous chapter – the alternatives are an instrumental birth (if it can safely done) or a caesar.

Elective caesars are deliberately scheduled before labour starts. Examples why we may book in an elective caesar include a baby in the breech position (bum in the pelvis instead of the head, meaning an attempted vaginal birth can be hazardous) or the mum has had caesars before (those who have had one previous caesar can choose to try again for a vaginal birth, or head straight for a caesar. There are pros and cons with either approach, which are discussed with the second-time mum during her pregnancy, and well in advance of birth).

What does the operating theatre look like?

For those having an emergency caesar, it may be a slightly disconcerting moment when they burst through the front doors of the operating suite and are wheeled in.

For starters, many operating suites are bathed in bright LED lighting (which, for some reason, are a stark white rather than a friendly, warm yellow glow). The brightness of the operating area will be a jolting visual contrast to the more dimly lit birth suite room where many hours were spent.

Theatre staff may descend on mum garbed in theatre scrubs, donned in masks, and wearing thin netting to cover their hair (though in December we may wear Christmas-y themed hair nets with cute festive symbols to try to make it fun). Adding to the medicalised feel, one of us will launch into a formal checklist: 'Do you have caps or crowns?' 'When was the last time you ate?' 'Do you have any allergies?' 'What's your favourite Jason Statham movie?'

The operating suite may cause a bit of a sensory overload, but be reassured that the theatre staff are really part of the same team with the singular aim of facilitating the safe arrival of babies. It's our day (and sadly, night) jobs and we are good at it. And we are all nice and friendly. So do your best to relax.

I thought it might be a nice idea to firstly get properly orientated by taking a tour around the operating room while a caesar is in action, but frozen in time. Just like the training modules in *The Matrix*.

Mum will be lying on the operating table in the middle of the room. I can't promise the most comfortable bedding (no plush mattress I'm afraid) but at least we can still offer a somewhat soft pillow (premium hospital grade quality, certified free of bedbugs. And you're welcome).

Loitering near the head of mum is the anaesthetist. Besides administering the spinal (or adding more drug into the epidural if one is in place) they watch over mum's vital signs throughout the operation – blood pressure, pulse rate, oxygen levels in her blood – keeping her safe. Often, they also provide comforting chitchat to calm mum's nerves. Most are great at it, but I can't vouch for the conversational skills of every anaesthetist (a few have a penchant to utter corny dad jokes so terrible they can make the surgeon feel like hurling mid-operation). There may also be an anaesthetic nurse nearby and they are a vital helping hand (they may also partake in the conversation if the topic interests them).

Next to the anaesthetist will be a vertical machine stack with fancy anaesthetic gadgetry: dials, nobs and a screen that provides a continuous read-out of mum's heart rate, blood pressure (as well as other vitals) for the anaesthetist's viewing pleasure. It's also rigged with a few gas canisters filled with the anaesthetic agents to put patients to sleep if needed (we hardly ever put women asleep for caesars).

Also seated in that now rather crowded corner near mum's head is someone very special – mum's nominated support person, who is often the partner. They can also freely chat with mum throughout the operation.

We are sensitive to the fact that some support people are nervous about venturing into the operation room. We understand some are squeamish: they avoid anything medical, never once streamed a medical drama and were already wary about coming along to the birth. Here are a few reassuring comments if this is you. There will be a strategically positioned drape running upwards from mum's chest towards the roof preventing you from seeing the operation. Also, you can step out any time you are overwhelmed. For those feeling light-headed and worried they may faint, there is ample time to vacate the operating suite to shake it off. So, don't worry. We will keep a caring eye on you too.

Let's now peel ourselves from this busy corner, take flight and hover over the operation, still frozen in time. There will be people standing along each side of mum performing the caesar. The primary surgeon will be on mum's right, adjacent to her abdomen (left-handed surgeons often stand on mum's left). Often, the primary surgeon will be no other than the obstetrician involved in the care throughout labour. This is great for the mum as she will have gotten to know them beforehand. Standing to mum's left and directly opposite the primary surgeon will be a surgical assistant. And next to the surgical assistant, standing alongside mum's legs will be a theatre scrub nurse with a tray of surgical instruments splayed out on a table next to them. They play a super important role, passing and collecting surgical instruments as they are requested. The surgeon needs tools handed to them quickly. I can vouch for the fact that having a skilled scrub nurse who can anticipate the tools I need before I ask for them makes an amazing difference. They really are an important member of the team (plus, having one who's fun to chat with is also a big bonus).

There may be a few others lurking about in the operating theatre. They include a theatre technician keeping a watchful eye over all the machines to ensure it's all in good working order; and a scrub scout who is on tap to fetch bits and pieces throughout the operation (such as more suture material or other surgical instruments from an adjoining room) and keeps count of instruments (so that the number of tools left in the belly after the operation equals exactly zero). You will probably hardly notice their fleet-footed presence.

Importantly, the familiar face of the kindly midwife who had been providing care during the long hours of labour will also be there. Seeing them in the operating theatre among all the new faces will be a most comforting sight.

Lastly, there may be a paediatric doctor in the room on standby to check over the newborn with the midwife. Both of them will be standing next to a resuscitation trolley in the theatre.

Our tour of the caesar 'in action' is at an end (please take the time to fill out the customer satisfaction survey on your way out through to the gift shop). Let's now un-pause and rewind to the moment when mum first arrives in the operating theatre.

How caesars are done

Before we start, we need to sort out anaesthesia so the caesar is a painless one. Most are done under regional anaesthesia – an epidural or spinal anaesthetic – which we covered back in

Chapter 2. If there is already an epidural in place the anaesthetist 'tops it up' by injecting more drug through the epidural tube. If there isn't, the anaesthetist will usually opt for a spinal anaesthetic – a single shot injection of local anaesthetic into the lower back.

A general anaesthetic, where mum is put asleep, is used for around 6 per cent of caesars in Australia. This ballpark figure probably applies to many other countries too. Putting mum asleep certainly isn't our preference. For one, mum isn't awake to see bubs being born, which is a bummer. Also, though very safe, a general anaesthetic is marginally riskier to mum compared to epidurals and spinals. Reasons why we go for a general anaesthetic is because the mum requests it (some cannot bear the thought of being awake during an operation and we respect this), or the baby's fetal heart rate pattern on the CTG is so shockingly poor that we think delivering the baby is time critical because oxygen levels may be really low (for example, a sudden drop in the fetal heart rate that has stayed alarmingly slow and hasn't returned to the baseline speed for over 10 minutes – a clear 'red light' signal on the CTG). In this extremely emergent situation, we are worried about further serious injury that could befall the baby if we even waited the extra 10–15 minutes for a spinal anaesthetic to be performed. Putting women asleep is much faster: it can be done in minutes and we can rapidly get on with the caesar to deliver the dangerously imperilled baby.

Once pain relief is on board, we lie mum down and slot a catheter into her bladder if she doesn't have one. To decrease the risk of surgical infection we will inject antibiotics through the intravenous drip, gently swab out the vagina with some antiseptic solution and paint the abdominal skin with antiseptic wash (usually a hot pink colour). We then surround the area where we will soon operate with surgical drapes which cordons off a nice perimeter – the surgical field. Besides giving the operation a nice Hollywood-esque flare, the purpose of these sterile drapes is to reduce the risk of infection. As mentioned, a fold of drape near mum's chest extends skywards, providing a visual barrier to prevent mum and the support person seeing the operation.

We start by making a skin incision around 12–15 centimetres long, which is what's needed to accommodate the baby's head. This cut is two fingers breadth above the pubic bone, roughly parallel to the upper border of underwear (after full recovery, when everything has deflated the scar often sits nicely tucked within the underwear).

We then incise the loose, yellow fat layer directly beneath the skin (which varies considerably in thickness). Next, we slice through a white fibrous layer called the 'rectus sheath'. This important fibrous sheath wraps the core of our body like a corset and helps keep the abdominal area of our bodies relatively taut and tubular, preventing us from blowing out like soft, amorphous slugs (though I'm afraid the rectus sheath can't prevent the expansion of love handles because the layer of fat forming these grip-able formations is closer to the surface of the body than the rectus sheath). It's a weakening of this fibrous rectus sheath that gives rise to troublesome hernias that afflict many in later life (and helps pay for bespoke house renovations of surgeons skilled at fixing them).

We next find our way into the abdominal cavity. Here I wish to clear up a common misconception: we don't cut the 'ab' muscles (rectus abdominus muscles – aka the 'six packs', for those still able to locate them) to reach the baby. Instead, we locate a vertical space between the two straps of muscles and enter in between. In fact, the modern surgical approach to enter the abdomen for caesars cunningly avoids cutting any core body muscles whatsoever. This also means that two months after the caesar, there is no excuse preventing you from restarting your strict, daily stomach crunch routine. (I once performed a caesar on a lovely private patient who is a high-ranking black belt taekwondo master. At her six-week postnatal visit she reported feeling great and was back to her '800 a day' stomach crunch routine. I certainly didn't recommend such a hectic exercise routine. In fact, I might have preferred that she had taken it more easily straight after the op to allow the tissues to heal more before restarting such taxing pursuits, but she was just fine. Her fitness blew me away – I can state with certainty my personal cumulative stomach crunch tally over a decade barely reaches her weekly count. Wow.)

Upon entering the abdominal cavity, we arrive at the uterus. Sitting in front of the uterus is the bladder (pregnant women can attest to this: they spend many infuriating nights visiting the bathroom repeatedly because their oversized uterus taps on the bladder next to it which gives them the sensation to urgently do number ones). We may gently separate the bladder from the uterus and slide it clear of the operative zone. We do this because the top edge of the bladder is close to where we make the definitive uterine incision to reach the baby. If we do not slide it away, we may risk damaging it during the operation.

Finally, we are set to deliver the munchkin. It has been waiting inside for months and probably quite impatient to see what its parents look like (does daddy look like me?). It's probably also been itching to make a move from its watery, jet-black existence to nab prized real estate in mum and dad's warm bed. It has had a lot of time to hatch a plot to dodge the lonely Ikea cot pegged for them: via a cunning strategy of disciplined, non-stop nocturnal howling. Once ensconced between its parents, bubby knows it can snooze and snack throughout the night. Furthermore, once in the parental bed it can green light stage two of its nefarious masterplan: precision regurgitations to evict non-birth parent to the couch bed. If successful it may come with rich rewards: more space, having mummy all to itself, and discouraging impulsive acts that may spawn rival siblings. (Community notice – co-sleeping is not 100 per cent safe and is best avoided. Hence, I strongly recommend that you resist the little rascal's dastardly plans.)

We perform a horizontal incision (that is, orientated parallel to the upper border of underwear) on the uterine wall, 10 or so centimetres in length. We split open the layers of the uterine muscle to reach the baby. Once we get through the full thickness of the muscular layer of the uterus and breach the inner cavity, the next layer we encounter contains the placental membranes. They bulge out like a taut layer of glad wrap with fluid swirling underneath. We break the waters by piercing a hole in the membranes whereupon amniotic fluid gushes out (straw coloured, or green if there is meconium). We use a 'sucker' that hoovers up this fluid (some may spill into the abdominal cavity, but the body will absorb this over time). During the operation you may hear this sucker, which sounds uncannily similar to gurgle of the milk frother used by the baristas whipping up a delicious caffeinated hit. When you hear this, you should be excited to know that birth is mere moments away.

The primary surgeon shapes their right hand like a spatula, reaches under the baby's head and scoops it through the hole in the uterus and out the skin incision. The assistant will be pushing on the abdomen on the top of the uterus to help push the baby out.

Sometimes we may use forceps to lift the baby out of the uterus. If we do, it's a vastly different proposition to using forceps to deliver the baby via the vagina. We are just using the forceps as a tool to ease out the head – there's none of the risks of instrumental births we discussed in the last chapter (except perhaps minor marks on the face but they quickly fade).

If the caesar is being done because the baby is in the breech position (bum in the pelvis instead of the head) we will reach in and find a foot. We then locate the other foot and slide out the legs. Bum, body, arms and head then follows.

Many of us are happy for the dividing drape to be partially lowered while baby is coming out, just enough so that mum and the support person can witness the birth. They may not see the head coming out but can see the rest of the body slide out. And if they had kept the sex of the baby a secret, they will find out at this truly memorable moment. Some prefer not to have the drapes lowered to witness the birth and that's absolutely fine.

We can't pass baby over the dividing drape straight to mum's chest as this will risk contaminating the clean operative field. It is super important not to offer opportunistic infectious nasties an easy path to slide into mum's open abdominal cavity. Many of our vital organs lurk in this cave – guts, liver, spleen – and unauthorised entry by a superbug with mischievous inclinations is best avoided.

We will cut the cord and hand the newborn to the midwife or paediatric doctor standing behind the primary surgeon (we can do delayed cord clamping if that's needed, or requested). The baby will be taken to the resuscitation trolley for a check. If the baby is pink, moving and squawking we will swaddle it and take the precious little being over to mum without delay. We present the baby on the pillow right next to her face and the newborn can be held by the spouse or support person. An incredibly special moment (we will have tissues nearby).

Direct skin-to-skin is definitely possible while the caesar is in progress (it is best to make the request to the midwife in advance). The baby can be perched on mum's chest just under the drape, held steady by the support person.

Birth at a caesar can be an emotional experience that is every bit as special as a vaginal birth. I have a fond memory of a new mum tugging on my (bloodied) surgical gown by the end of the caesar thanking me and gushing how she loved every second of it.

And just like a vaginal birth, within moments of the bundle of (anticipated) joy arriving, the emotional ambience drastically shifts. Once baby is handed to mum and support person, overwhelming relief often replaces tense anticipation that mounted over the many hours of labour. This often happens well before the operation has even finished. The theatre can suddenly become a jolly place to be.

Once the uterus is empty the anaesthetist will inject oxytocin drugs to contract the uterus, just like we do at a vaginal birth. The surgeon then delivers the placenta (a very easy thing to do as we have direct access to the inside of the uterus), confirms that the uterus is empty (no daggy bits of placenta or placental membranes left clinging onto the inner walls of the uterine cavity), then stitches closed the uterine incision. Most of the bleeding from a caesar comes from the cut edge of the uterine incision. Trickling starts with the first cut; bleeding continues while the incision remains open and only stops when we have securely sewn it up. This means we don't muck about when we open and close the uterus.

After stitching the uterus and checking that the incision site has completely stopped bleeding, we simply close the layers of the abdominal wall that we opened to reach baby. Besides the uterus the other important layers that we need to close are the fibrous rectus sheath and the skin. We may also put in a few stitches in the fat layer prior to closing the skin. Many of us will stitch the skin using a fancy technique that completely buries the suture material (which dissolve by themselves).

The time it takes to enter the abdomen and birth the baby is quick. On average, the baby appears within 5–10 minutes of commencing the caesar. Sewing up the layers takes longer, around 20–35 minutes on average (it can take longer for caesars that are a little more difficult). This means from the first cut on the skin to full skin closure, most caesars take roughly 30–45 minutes.

Once the baby is out, mum may find the rest of the caesar passing by with little notice. Most women won't be mulling over the curious predicament of being awake with a completely numb abdomen and their abdominal cavity wide open. Often, they are too busy engaged in pressing mummy matters, such as gazing lovingly at her new baby and exchanging tender whispers with her support person. The anaesthetist and the anaesthetic nurse standing close by may earnestly reassure the new parents that their baby is indeed the most beautiful they have ever seen during their entire practising career *(cough)*. The surgeons may also partake in the social chatter, perhaps enquiring whether the couple had yet settled on a name from their shortlist that best suits the adorable face (experienced obstetricians have literally done thousands of caesars. We can safely chat while we sew).

And that's all there is to it. Mum can then wave goodbye to her new friends in the operation room as she is wheeled to the recovery area, where she rests for half an hour or so. Support person, baby and midwife usually shuffle off to the ward, and mum will join them soon. Some hospitals are able to accommodate both support person and new baby in the recovery area so they can be with mum, but you will probably need to request this ahead of time. If your health service is unable to accommodate this, please go with that – with the profound relief that it's all over, mums often fall into a deep slumber as soon as they reach the recovery area anyway (and they richly deserve a hearty snooze). Then soon enough, mum will be spirited away to the postnatal ward where she can cuddle her delicious miracle at will.

Pain relief after a caesar

An irritating myth widely circulated is that recovery from a caesar is a horrifying six-week test of endurance. A pain-ridden existence where even venturing out of bed is an agonising saga. This is just not true.

Recovery after most caesars is straightforward. And quite quick. With good pain management, discomfort can be kept to a minimum the moment mum is wheeled out of the operating room. By about three weeks most will not require any pain relief meds at all. They are just freely doing their thing. And perhaps pondering whether they are allowed to drive (for my private patients the answer is yes, but only if they are off all pain relief meds and their car insurance policies allow them to. But I also ask them to be sensible – keep drives short for the first six weeks after the op. No lengthy road trips criss-crossing the country plains).

Strong opiate-based painkillers such as endone and oxycontin will be offered over the first few days after a caesar. These are important to take as they are the strongest oral painkillers we've got. Pain control is paramount.

The opiate-based painkillers can cause some women to feel spaced out. This doesn't always happen and a (lucky) few actually get a sense of euphoria. Even if mum feels a little spacey, she should continue taking them because adequate pain relief is really important. The need for regular doses of strong opiate pain meds drops away within days after the caesar. And within a week (certainly two) more conventional meds such as paracetamol and ibuprofen (which do not make people feel woozy) will be more than enough to keep the pain at bay.

I lament the fact that some women are left to endure too much pain after a caesar because their post-operative pain has not been managed well. It is so avoidable and unnecessary. My strong advice for those who have just had a caesar is this: stay on top of the pain. Don't be shy to ask for painkillers if you need them and anticipate the need for more before the pain escalates. If women find themselves frozen in bed with pain with the thought of moving terrifying them, they are not only underdone but have fallen way behind their pain medication requirements.

They should load up and get comfy so they can resume the happy motherly task of baby bonding, wince free.

The rest of recovery after a caesar

The day of the caesar is mainly R and R in bed. A moment to catch breath and get acquainted with baby. However, even on the day of the operation women can shuffle about once the anaesthetic wears off and have a nice warm shower.

Mums can eat on the day of the surgery (some surgeons prefer to keep mum fasted until there is evidence their bowels are gurgling, but not me). I do suggest keeping the first meals light and resist going the full steak, chips 'n' gravy as the first meal. I had a delightful private patient who ravenously launched into crispy hot chips within hours after her caesar. She was privileged to witness the deep-fried treat reappear all over her gown in a far less appetising form.

And for sure, mums can breastfeed after a ceasar. We strongly encourage it. Midwives at the hospital have skills to teach women how to breastfeed. For those who are having difficulties, lactation consultants are available at many units to provide expert assistance. Needless to say, all the meds we give for pain relief are safe with breastfeeding.

On the first day after the caesar (after the first night), women will find they can shuffle about quite a bit. They will still need strong painkillers taken regularly. Their urinary catheter and intravenous drip can be removed, meaning they are entirely 'tube' free. If they haven't done so already, it's nice to replace the (alarmingly airy) regulation hospital gown with their personal nightgown.

By day two after the caesar many will already feel they have turned a corner. They are more comfortable and moving about freely. They can sit on the couch to rest and breastfeed rather than defaulting to the bed. The new mum may even start venturing outside their room and waddle about the ward, proudly displaying their new centre of gravity.

Unless specific medical issues arise, most women will be ready for home after a three-night stay (some hospitals offer even earlier discharge). As they step out the door, they should take a prescription to collect more pain relief medications to take at home, which they gradually wean themselves off over ensuing weeks. As mentioned, most will stop all their pain meds by the third week. A fortunate few will have even comfortably dispensed with the painkillers within a week of arriving home (but remember that there is no rush to stop the pain relief meds. In fact, do freely take them until the pain has gone).

It is definitely true that there is more to recover from after a caesar compared to a straightforward vaginal birth, especially those having their second or third natural birth. In terms of recovery for the mother, an uncomplicated vaginal birth is the best path to take. But if a caesar is needed, be reassured that with good pain management it can be made a comfortable road. Within weeks most women return to daily activities unhindered.

The risks of having a caesar

Although a caesar is an operation, it's a very safe one. An emergency caesar is a smidgen riskier, but on the whole it's still very safe.

There are some risks to know about. All operations incur a bleeding risk (so does a vaginal birth, as you may recall). Heavier than usual blood losses happen for caesars where the cut muscle edges of the uterine incision (made to get baby out) bleeds profusely while it remains open. The bleeding only ceases when the incision is stitched shut. How briskly the cut edge of uterine muscles bleed between caesar to caesar varies widely, and we can't know who will bleed more heavily until we make the cut. Except that, in general, caesars after a long labour bleed more briskly than elective caesars for pregnancies that never went into labour.

Another reason why we may encounter heavier losses is because there are tears that extend beyond the original horizontal uterine incision we made to birth the baby. They arise on occasion while we are delivering the baby. If they appear, it means we need to fix the tear as well as the original uterine incision. Tears occur more often for caesars done after women have been labouring a long time.

Of course, we will get on top of any tears to uterine muscles to stop the bleeding; however, occasionally they are surgically challenging. And while we are stitching, blood losses mount until all repairs are done.

Tears arise the most often for caesars done when the cervix is fully dilated. There are a few reasons for this. A long first stage followed by a long period of active pushing renders the uterine muscles pretty fragile, making it more easily torn. Secondly, the head is wedged more deeply in the pelvis and can be very challenging for the obstetrician to scoop out, especially when compared to an elective caesar where the head is still perched high in the abdomen and within easy reach. Lifting the head out of the pelvis can sometimes be a struggle and cause tearing of the uterine muscle, which then requires expert repair.

Consequently, fully dilated caesars are one of the more difficult procedures we do as obstetricians. We can perform them safely, but while we are doing a caesar at full dilatation there just may be less chatter coming from us over the drape compared to when we are leisurely doing an elective caesar.

The consequence of excessive blood loss is that mum may be anaemic after the operation (lower than normal red blood cells in her body), revealed by a blood test done after the procedure. If the anaemia is minor, which is most often the case, all that's needed is for mum to take iron tablets for the ensuing weeks after the birth. This helps replenish the red blood cells lost at the caesar (iron is an essential ingredient to make new red blood cells). For more serious bleeding, mum may end up more severely anaemic after the operation. If the haemoglobin (red blood cell) levels in her blood are very low, we may need to offer an iron transfusion or a blood transfusion. The risk of needing a blood transfusion after a caesar is around 1 per cent (it's probably a little higher for caesars done at full dilatation).

A wound infection is a risk after any operation. Luckily, if it happens most are minor, discovered as a redness somewhere along the skin incision. Sometimes, a few centimetres of the skin incision gapes open and is moistened by a small amount of straw-coloured fluid (aka pus).

Keep in mind that wound infections can set in any time over the next few weeks after the operation. Hence, mum and her partner should take a glance now and then at the skin incision after they arrive home. And if they suspect that there is an infection brewing, they should quickly get it checked out because early treatment is key to staying out of trouble – in most cases, a course of oral antibiotics and splashing antiseptic wash onto the site of the infection will solve the problem. Within days the redness goes away, the wound dries up and gaps in the skin seal up.

More serious infections causing the mother to become quite unwell can happen but are infrequent, troubling around 1 per cent of all caesars. Such infections typically affect the wound site, but can also arise in odd spots, like the bladder. Mum may need to be re-admitted to hospital to receive a few days of intravenous antibiotics. This is indeed a most unwelcome development, but if it happens most maternity hospitals allow the new baby to room in.

Infections and excessive bleeding (which we have just discussed) are the main risks of a caesar to know about. They are uncommon but they do occur. Here we will now turn other complications that are rarer – the risk for any of them is 0.5 per cent or less – but they are rather more serious if they do happen.

A deep vein thrombosis is a risk after any operation (in fact, it is a risk after childbirth). This is where a blood clot forms deep within the calf muscle on the lower leg, lodged in one of the deep veins. The danger in having such a stagnant lump of blood clot sitting in a leg vein is that a fragment of the clot can break away and travel through mum's circulation to her lungs. There, it can block off blood vessels which can be a very dangerous thing as it interferes with the lung's ability to absorb oxygen. This is clearly not good and can even be fatal.

But don't worry. The risk of this is already very low and we do things to reduce it further. We get women on their feet and moving about soon after the caesar to keep blood flowing through the calf veins and preventing it from stagnating. We may put on tight 'compression stockings' on mum's legs to further discourage blood in the calf to clot (sadly, they're usually an unimaginative stark white in keeping with the sterile ambience of hospitals. And they can get a touch sticky during sweltering summers). We may also give tiny injections of a blood thinner over the first few days after the caesar which also decreases the risk of clots forming. By doing all this, the risk of a deep vein thrombosis after a caesar is minimised to one in several hundred cases or less.

Any operation in the abdomen incurs a very small risk that the surgeon inadvertently injures a neighbouring structure inside the abdominal cavity. The bladder is closest and is most at risk. However, most inadvertent bladder injuries can be easily repaired and will fully heal with no ongoing issues. Damage to other structures – such as the ureters (long tubes that join the kidneys to the bladder and skirt along the sides of the uterus) or loops of bowels – can be more rather more serious. Happily, accidental injuries to these important structures are rare. And they can be repaired if they happen, though fixing injuries to the ureter or bowels can be very involved.

Requesting an elective caesar rather than labouring as the birth plan

A small number of women request a caesar as their preferred path to birth their first baby. They may be a little nervous about asking for this because they are worried that well-meaning friends and family may view this request dimly. And judge her. The mum-to-be may have even confided these thoughts to a close friend only to be blasted by an aggressive response, as if they were being talked off a ledge. This is unfortunate.

What do I think? As I noted from the beginning, I am as neutral as Switzerland. For a small number of women, it is a valid choice. I will provide some objective facts and leave it to the expectant mum to decide what is best for her.

So here are the pros and cons of a caesar done because of 'maternal request', and in the absence of a specific medical reason. Offered here so that women can make their own informed decision. Of course, anyone seriously thinking about this should have a long chat about it with their own obstetric team during one of their antenatal visits, well ahead of birth.

Some people might be riled by this statement: a caesar is the safest path for baby. This is because, as you well know by now, the uterine contractions that occur during labour can be stressful for babies. An elective caesar bypasses this entirely. However, I would quickly add that modern obstetric management can facilitate extremely safe attempts at vaginal birth. Hence, I most certainly do not advocate heading for a caesar because of the miniscule risk to babies arising from the stress of labour.

A meaty pro is that a caesar comprehensively protects the mum's pelvic floor from any risk of birth trauma to the pelvis. It entirely removes the risk of a third-degree tear (a tear in the anal sphincter muscle) – indeed, any vaginal tearing. But I will quickly add that tearing for a majority of vaginal births is small, easily mended, and often equates to a lesser amount tissue injury than a caesar itself. However, the caesar allows women to sidestep the roughly 5–10 per cent risk (for first-time mums) of a rather more serious injury to the pelvic floor which has a protracted recovery time (a small proportion of these cases will have ongoing symptoms that are permanent).

There are cons. The first is obvious: the mum will incur all the risks of having an operation that we just discussed. Secondly, performing successive caesarean sections (third, fourth, fifth repeat caesars) can get progressively more challenging because there can be more and more tissue scaring every time we repeat the operation. If there is significant or dense scaring, the tissues we are operating on may be distorted, making the procedure more difficult. Very occasionally, if we find a repeat caesarean section immensely challenging to do, we may gently ask the mum to think twice before falling pregnant again. This usually only becomes an issue when women have reached their third or fourth repeat caesar (fourth or fifth child). Also, whether dense scarring appears with subsequent caesars varies enormously between women.

While we are on this topic, I would like to quash a rumour that there is a hard limit of three caesars for everyone. This is untrue – I have safely performed many third and fourth repeat caesars. Even a fifth repeat.

Finally, there is a small risk that is worth knowing about: a rare obstetric complication called a placenta accreta. This is where the placenta embeds low down in the uterine cavity and gets stuck in the scar of the uterine wall made from the previous caesar. They are a big problem as the placenta won't separate from the uterus after the baby is birthed. The placenta is plain stuck and the mum will usually end up with heavy bleeding and a hysterectomy. Losing the uterus means no further births are possible. Placenta accretas are very rare, but the risk rises from one in many thousands for those who never had a caesar, to one in a few hundred for those who have had three or more caesars (elevating the risk from rare to very uncommon).

A frequent reason why some ask for a caesar is that they are petrified of the (anticipated) pain in labour. If this is the pervading concern then I suggest trying for a vaginal birth, but to request an early epidural as a centrepiece of the birth plan. An early epidural may be a great a solution for women who deeply fear the (anticipated) pain of labour, and avoids the need to head straight for a caesar.

Requesting a primary caesar – done for maternal request and in the absence of a specific medical need – is really anticipating fate's roll of the die. It will have been a fantastic decision if the labour was destined for nasty birth trauma to the baby or mother. But if one's destiny was a straightforward vaginal birth (with a tiny tear that heals quickly, or no tear at all), this would have been, by far, the best outcome. Besides having next to nothing to heal from, they can look forward to similarly smooth births for all future pregnancies instead of consecutive operations (after one normal vaginal birth, the chances of having another one next time are high). By having a caesar before labour even begins, we'll never know.

There is no doubt that the caesarean section has prevented the premature demise of untold numbers of babies that might otherwise have failed to take their first gasp. And saved huge numbers of babies from suffering major injury from a wayward birth that would have otherwise wreaked serious, permanent disabilities such as cerebral palsy and developmental delays.

I hope this chapter has been enlightening, whether or not a caesar will be part of your future birth experience. Yes, it's an abdominal operation, but a very safe procedure that is commonly done. There are risks – some of the rarer ones are serious – but most caesars occur without a hitch where all traces of the operation (except a faint tell-tale scar) vanish within weeks.

Here I might I take this opportunity to congratulate you. By making it all the way to this part of the book, I reckon you now know far more about the road to birth than most others approaching this auspicious event.

I hope this inside knowledge will do all the things for you that I said it might back in the Introduction. It will suit you up for the big day, and serve as a shield to protect you from the very human trait of being terrified because you don't understand what's going on.

As I mentioned from the outset, I worry about how we can hastily spoon information into women in the throes of labour once it's apparent that a caesar or instrumental birth is required. Now you have boned up for the big day, I am hoping a lack of informed consent for anything that birth throws at you won't be your problem.

Finally, it is my hope that learning about all the possible paths to birth – including the ones that you (or the person you are supporting) ultimately do *not* take – will further enrich your birth experience.

Recap: Birth by caesarean section

1. Just like for instrumental births, the main reasons why caesars are done are fetal distress or arrested labour. It's the only option to expedite birth in the first stage of labour. It's also done during the second stage of labour if it is deemed too dangerous to deliver the baby via an instrumental birth (mainly because the baby has not descended low enough down the birth canal).

2. Most are done with an epidural or spinal anaesthetic. This means mum can be awake and watch the important moment when baby is born. It is uncommon to do caesars while mum is asleep.

3. Mum can have a support person sitting close by. Besides being privileged to bear witness to a memorable occasion, this person is bestowed the earnest responsibility of bringing an adequately charged phone (or camera) to take photos.

4. The concept of a caesar is pretty simple. We make sideways incisions on the skin, fat and a fibrous layer in the abdominal wall. We then enter the abdominal cavity in between the abdominal muscles (but we do not cut them). We perform a sideways cut through the uterus to deliver the baby. After this, we stitch up the layers we opened, starting with the womb.

5. Once it's apparent that bubby is breathing, pink and well, the little bundle will be quickly taken to the parents. And held very close to mum's head for the rest of the caesar. Direct skin-to-skin during the caesar is even possible (though I suggest the request is made in advance).

6. Recovery after a caesar is often straightforward and quicker than most imagine. With good pain management the new mum can be kept very comfortable from the outset. She can be shuffling about on the day of her caesar and moving about freely the day after. Most will be off all pain meds by around three weeks after the operation.

7. It's a very safe procedure but there are some risks. Like vaginal births, there can be significant blood loss via heavy bleeding, but this can be countered with iron tablets, iron transfusion or (on occasion) a blood transfusion. Although infections can happen, most are minor and can be fixed with antibiotic tablets. Uncommonly, some infections are more serious and require hospital admission and intravenous antibiotics. Much rarer complications include deep vein thrombosis (a blood clot in the calves) or an accidental injury to neighbouring structures in the abdomen (which can be mended but can be very involved).

8. Please bear in mind that for those who end up with one, caesars are very safe and recovery is often quick. Mum can be awake to see her bubby being born, she can most definitely pick up her baby after the operation, she can breastfeed and will be up on her feet very soon after the operation.

Farewell and good luck with the day of birth

Thanks for your company. I've enjoyed being your personal guide on this rather unique tour. Securely fastened to our seats, in the safety of the tour bus and gazing out the window, we might have experienced a few things that are quite new to you.

Now I know it sucked that this was an educational trip, not a 'get sloshed and have fun' vacation. To make it 'fun' I tried to be as engaging as Pietro, the Italian guide on the bus during my own Trafalgar tour of Italy (circa 2003). Like Pietro, I hope I managed to keep you entertained with the odd quirky historical fact. Or by my odd attempts at humour. Or just by being odd.

No doubt this holiday was noticeably different to your more languid car trip up the coast last year. For starters we had to patiently ripen the cervix to even get the holiday started (generally not a feature of most vacations). And once we were finally off and away it was certainly not a quick, smooth ride. Instead, it was treacherous. We sweltered through a long journey to traverse the first stage of labour. This part of the itinerary dribbled on far longer than you may have thought when you glanced over the glossy brochure. And it was rough going; no sleep, no devices (remember?). Even visits to the loo were a struggle. And being made to wear those airy gowns on the bus was weird.

We all watched with consternation as the road got bumpy. And we dodged some alarming potholes. The bus stalled for a bit (apologies, I will speak with the manager) and we had to rev up the motor by adding some fresh juice to get us on the move again. We suddenly found the driver manoeuvring the bus slowly. When we all peered out the window we discovered why; we found ourselves staring at CTG fetal heart rate patterns fluttering across the sky, fluxing between amber and green signals. I felt the breath of anticipation of the entire tour group on my neck while I deliberated with the driver whether it may be safer to open the hatch on the roof of the bus, empty the vehicle and end the trip right then and there.

But by carefully controlling the speed of the bus and not overly stressing the system, the highly experienced driver got us to the second stage (thanks, driver). Though once we arrived, we were all made to work hard. The tour group (already grousing over the discomfort of this year's supposed 'getaway') did not anticipate being ordered off the bus to crowd behind it and push. But that we did. I pushed. The driver pushed. We all pushed. And pushed. For a full hour and a half. It was such hard work (the bus was hardly budging with every heave) and many of us were drenched by the end of it.

But it was all worth it: for we all witnessed the incredible marvel of birth.

We breathed a sigh of relief when the shoulders emerged with ease. The placenta quickly followed. There was a fleeting moment of high drama (which holiday doesn't have one of those?) when the bleeding became rather brisk. Happily, it settled promptly after a flurry of activity (phew, bleeding is never good, especially while on vacation). Just a few small repairs to mend the undercarriage of the bus and we were off again.

And before we knew it, we arrived home.

Sadly, the long-distance trip messed with our body clocks quite a bit. We all just knew it would be months before we ever get to sleep through the night without waking. But that didn't matter as we got to take home the most precious of souvenirs – one that sure beats a snowdome of Big Ben, the Eiffel Tower (I think) or the Sydney Harbour Bridge.

The trip – a dress rehearsal really – is now over. Thanks again for your company. I hope you have learnt a heap and that the travels we have taken together will help make the birth you will soon have – or are soon to witness – a wonderful, positive experience. An event you will long cherish as one of the most memorable days of your life.

I do warmly wish you the very best for the real event.